HOMEOPATHIC MEDICINE AND SYMPTOMS

By the Same Author

Understanding Homeopathy: A Handbook (2017) published by Good Times Books Pvt. Ltd., New Delhi.

About the Author

Dr. Arun Lata Srivastava, born in Sitapur, Uttar Pradesh, has been practicing Homeopathy since 1996 in Lucknow, purely on charitable basis. She is helping poor and lower strata of society by giving them free consultation and medicines.

Most of the time she keeps busy in National seminars and conferences to facilitate Homeopathy all around the country. Apart from above aspect of life she has an other personality in literacy taste too. She is author of several story books, poetry collection and novel in Hindi.

HOMEOPATHIC MEDICINE AND SYMPTOMS

Arun Lata Srivastava

CONCEPT PUBLISHING COMPANY PVT. LTD.
NEW DELHI - 110 059

ISBN: 978-93-5594-654-6 (HB)
ISBN: 978-93-5594-655-3 (PB)

First Published 2024

Published and Printed by

Concept Publishing Company Pvt. Ltd.
A/15-16, Commercial Block, Mohan Garden
New Delhi-110059 (India)
T: +91-11-41101460
E: publishing@conceptpub.com, *W*: www.conceptpub.com

Cataloging in Publication--Courtesy: D.K. Agencies (P) Ltd. <docinfo@dkagencies.com>

Srivastava, Arun Lata, author.
Homeopathic medicine and symptoms / Arun Lata Srivastava.
pages cm
ISBN 9789355946546 (HB)
ISBN 9789355946553 (PB)

1. Homeopathy--Materia medica and therapeutics. I. Title.

LCC RX601.S65 2024 | DDC 615.532 23

Dedicated to
My Father
Late Sri Sunder Lal Srivastava

Preface

This is evidently a book on HOMEO THERAPEUTICS. I have helpfully introduced quite a number of subjects which are calculated to enable the general readers to grasp the main text far more intelligently than it would have been otherwise possible.

Profoundly, clear-cut symptoms of remedies incorporated under Therapeutics. At all events, every endeavor has been made to make the work immensely practical and perspicuously guiding.

The book has been written in pleasing style aiming at the requirements of the students, laymen, as well as the general practitioners.

Arun Lata Srivastava

Acknowledgements

During the writing, many people have helped me to make my task complete easily. I, therefore, acknowledge the contribution of every person. First of all my patients, friends and relatives swho have demanding the book which could help them to understand the Homeopathic medicines according to symptoms. First of all, I acknowledge luminaries and emimnt author Herrings, Farrington, J.H. Clarks, H.C. Allen, Boericke, Bhattacharya, Bhanja, Ghosh and many more who have contributed their knowledge and experience through writing books on Homeopathy.

I am also thankful to my husband Dr. Kamal Kumar Srivastava who has rendered congenial environment to write this book.

I am thankful to reverend Dr. Girish Gupta and Dr. Arvind, who shared their experiences. This paved me courage and confidence. I am thankful to my father Late Sri Sunder Lal Srivastava who had vision in me doing something for Society.

Lastly, I am thankful to Mr. Ashish Kashyap who rendered full domestic help whenever needed, in order to let me **free to complete this herculean task.**

Arun Lata Srivastava

Contents

Preface vii
Acknowledgements ix
• Abscess 1
• Acidity 2
• Alcoholism 3
• Amenorrhoea Suppression of Menses 4
• Anaemia 4
• Angina Pectoris, Breast-Pang 5
• Anus, Affections of 6
• Apoplexy 7
• Appendicitis 8
• Asphyxia-Apparent Death (Gas Poisoning) 10
• Arthritis-Gout 10
• Asthma 12
• Bedsores 14
• Bites and Stings 14
• Boils 17
• Bone Diseases 18
• Brain-Fag 19
• Bronchitis, Acute 19
• Bronchitis, Chronic 20
• Burns 21
• Cancer 22
• Carbuncle 24
• Cataract 25

- Cholera 26
- Cholera Infantum 28
- Colic 29
- Colic of Infants 30
- Constipation 30
- Convulsions 32
- Corns on Sole of Feet 33
- Coruplency (Great Obesity) 33
- Coryza 34
- Cough 35
- Cramps 37
- Dandruff 38
- Dentition 38
- Diabetes Mellitus 39
- Diarrhoea 40
- Diphtheria 42
- Dysentery 43
- Dysmenorrhoea (Painful Periods) 45
- Dyspepsia, Indigestion 46
- Dengue (Breakbone Fever) 48
- Earache-Otalgia 51
- Eczema 51
- Enuresis 53
- Epilepsy 54
- Epistaxis 56
- Erysipelas (Lymph Nodes) 58
- Eyelids, Affections or Swelling of Eyelids 59
- Face, Pimples on, Acnes 61
- Fainting 61
- False Pains 62
- Fever (Simple) 63
- Fistula 63
- Foreign Bodies in Tissues Etc. 64
- Fractures 65
- Frostbite, Chilblain 66
- Gall-Stone Colic 67
- Gangrene 68

- Gastralgia 69
- Gastritis 70
- Gastric Ulcer, Duodenal Ulcer 72
- Glands, Affections of 73
- Glaucoma 75
- Gleet 75
- Goitre 76
- Gums, Affections of 77
- Hamatemesis (Vomiting of Blood) 78
- Haemoptysis 79
- Haematuria (Haemorrhage Urinary Organs) 80
- Head, Congestion of Blood to 81
- Headache 82
- Hearing, Defects of 85
- Hair, Falling of 86
- Heart, Palpitation of 87
- Haemorrhoids, Piles 88
- Hernia 89
- Hiccough 90
- Hoarseness, Aphonia 91
- Hydrocele 92
- Hydrocephalus 92
- Hysteria 94
- Impotence 95
- Influenza 97
- Injuries 98
- Insomnia, Sleeplessness 99
- Intermittent Fever 101
- Jaundice 104
- Kidney, Affections of 105
- Lactation Derangements 107
- Leprosy 108
- Leucorrhoea, Whites 109
- Liver, Affections of (L. Cirrhosis) 111
- Lochial Discharge, Derangement in 113
- Locomotor Ataxa 114
- Lumbago, Backache 116

- Mastitis 118
- Masturbation 119
- Measles 120
- Meningitis 122
- Menorrhagia, Metrorrhagia 123
- Mental Derangement 123
- Metritis 125
- Miscarriage, Abortion 125
- Morning Sickness 127
- Mumps, Parotitis 128
- Nails, Affections of 129
- Nervousness 129
- Neuralgia 130
- Night-Blindness 132
- Nightmare 132
- Ophthalmia 133
- Orchitis 136
- Otorrhoea 136
- Abscess of Meatus 138
- Ovaries, Affections of 138
- Paralysis 140
- Photophobia 143
- Phthisis (Tuberculosis of Lungs) 144
- Plague 150
- Pleurisy 151
- Pneumonia 152
- Polypus 155
- Post-Partum Haemorrhage 156
- Puerperal Fever 157
- Puerperal Mental Derangements 158
- Remittent Fever 159
- Renal Colic 160
- Rheumatism 162
- Ringworm 165
- Salivation 166
- Scabies 167
- Sciatica 168

- Sea-Sickness, Rain-Sickness 171
- Smallpox 172
- Snuffles 174
- Sore Nipples 175
- Sore Mouth, Apthae 175
- Sore Throat, Pharingitis 176
- Spermatorrhea and Pollutions 178
- Stammering 180
- Stye 181
- Sunstroke 182
- Syphilis 183
- Tetanus and Trismus 187
- Tetanus Neonatorum 189
- Tongue, Discolouration of 189
- Tonsilitis Quinsy 190
- Tooth, Decaying of 192
- Toothache 192
- Tumours 196
- Typhoid Fever 197
- Ulcers 200
- Urinary Ailment 202
- Uterus, Prolapsus Displacement of 203
- Varicose Veins 204
- Vertigo Giddiness 205
- Vision, Defects, Loss, or Impairment of 206
- Vomiting and Nausea 207
- Warts 208
- Whitlow, Felons 209
- Whooping Cough 210
- Worm, Affections of 212
- Marasmus 214
- Rickets, Rachitis 215

Name of Medicines 217

ABSCESS

Therapeutics Leading Indications

Acon: Swelling very red and shining with burning in with dry hot skin.

Bell: Bright redness, *esp*. Radiating redness; much burn parts feel dry, hot. Decided aggravation from slight; Mammary, hepatic or rather glandular abscesses.

Merc-s: Use it only in the first stage of suppuration to promote discharge of pus. Suppuration slow forms in cavities which burn and sting. Bloody pus. Worse at night.

Hepar: May be given in high potency to preview suppuration before the opening of an abscess, particulars when there in throbbing. Here Hepar 200 has the effect either absorbing or opening an abscess (our experience). Pus which may be bloody smell like old cheese.

Silica: After discharge of pus has taken place, for some time and then give Silica. (say 30th) which has effect of healing the suppurating abscess. When abscess speedily, points, but pus is too scanty. Very useful when fistulous opening has formed. In chronic and when discharge is tardy, long-continued.

***

Arsen: When an abscess threatens to become gangrenous; great debility. Parts burn like fire.

Bryon: In the beginning when the part is very shining or very pale and hard, and feels stitching pains aggravated by slightest motion.

Rhus-Tox: Abscess of axillary and parotid glands.

Sulph: Continual tendency to relaps. Chronic abscess. In some cases, when Silicia, ceases to act after some time, a dose or two of sulphur, it interpolated, reactive energies of the system are then aroused and Silicia then Silicia enabled to cure the case.

ACIDITY

Therapeutics, Leading Indications

Carb-V: Sour risings after a meal. Burning in stomach; excessive flatulence. Much offensive flatus.

Iris: Great burning distress in stomach; sour vomiting. Burning in throat and esophagus, sometimes extending down to stomach; acid risings. (In the light of my experience, it is a great remedy in acidity, which is very often overlooked.)

Nux-v: Heartburn. Sour eructation's. *Pressure in stomach after meal.

Robin: *Acidity worse at night on lying down. Vomiting of intensely sour fluid which sets the teeth on edge.

Sulph-ac: Heartburn with sour eructation's that set the teeth on edge. Weak and exhausted. Chronic acidity.

***

China: When abdomen feels full and tight.

Lyco: Acid gnawing in stomach. Constant sense of Fermentation in stomach.

After-Pains

Unless severe and long lasting, there is nothing abnormal in after-pain, it being required to expel the blood clots and other foreign matters retained in uterus.

Therapeutics Leading Indications

Bell: Severe bearing down pains, as if contents of pelvis wounds protrude. *Slightest jar hurts her.

Cup-m: Most distressing crimpy pains, *esp.* in women who have borne many children.

Gels: Uterus feels as if squeezed by a hand.

Nux-v: Desire to go to stool with every pains.

Puls: Pains too long and too violent; worse towards evening. Mild, tearful disposition.

Secale: Long-continued and intense pains; lochia thin and offensive; feels cold but does not wish covering. Thin, scrawny feeble women.

ALCOHOLISM

Therapeutics Leading Indications

Angelica: "In fifteen drop doses of the tincture, three times a day, has caused disgust for liquor." (Raue)

Arsen: Seriously diseased by overuse of alcohol. Great restlessness, anxiety, fear of death.

Bell: Imagines he sees ghosts, hideous faces etc.; wants to run away from them; indistinct speech.

Calc-c: When Bell fails to cure or to effect more improvement. On closing eyes sees horrible visions. Constant fear of going crazy. Long sleeplessness.

Gels: Insomnia after abuse of alcoholic drinks.

Nux-v: Frequently helpful, gastric derangements, Awakens tired and weak.

Opium: In old sinners with thoroughly broken-down constitution; when asleep breathing is torturous; tremor.

Sulph-ac: Drunkard on his "last lege"; pale, shriveled, emaciated; cold; stomach will not tolerate any food; *sensation of internal trembling (outwardly no trembling); weak and exhausted. Hering says that one part of sulphuric acid with three parts of alcohol, if taken thrice daily in 10 to 15 drops doses for a period of three or four weeks, subdues craving for alcohol.

AMENORRHOEA SUPPRESSION OF MENSES

Therapeutics Leading Indications

Acon: Suppression of menses after fright. In young girl of a full plethoric habit who lead a sedentary life.

Apis: Young girls who are very busy and restless by doing nothing right, constantly changing occupation; awkward, lets things fall owing to muscular incoordinations.

Bell: Bearing-down pain in hypogastrium as if menses would appear; rush of blood to head.

Bryon: Vicarious menstruation; bleeding of nose when menses should appear (Bell., Puls.).

Calc-c: Caused by working in water; fat, indolent women cold, damp feet. Beginning of phthisis.

Gels: Sensation of heaviness in uterine region with drowsiness and apathy; aching across sacrum as if menses should appear.

Kali-C: Particularly efficacious at age of puberty. Stiffiness and pain in small of back. When Nat-m. fails although indicated, Kali-c. will bring on menses.

Puls: Caused by getting feet wet; constant chilliness even in a warm room; vicarious nosebleed. Often Graph. and Sulph. Come into play after failure of Puls.

Conium: Menses stops by putting hands in cold water. But effects of suppressed menses. Tremulous weakness. Breasts soar, hard and painful before and during menstruation (Lac-c., Kali-c.).

Rhus-t: After getting wet in rains.

Sepia: *Esp.* in chronic amenorrhoea. Scanty, irregular menstruation; dingy spots on face.

ANAEMIA

Therapeutics Leading Indications

Alumin: Anaemia in young girls at puberty; menses pale and secanty. Abnormal craving for indigestible substances.

China: Caused by loss of animal fluids, as from hemorrhage, loss of semen, long continued diarrhoea, leucorrhoea etc.

Calc-p. With too early menses. Thin, spare subjects; pale, waxy skin. Tendency to perspiration. With chronic gonorrhea.

Kali-c. Anaemia with debility; great tendency to perspire, backache.

Puls: Constant feeling of chilliness and still feeling better in open air. With menstrual and uterine disorders, After abuse of iron and quinine.

***

Arsen: Pernicious anaemia; excessive debility; odomatous swellings.

Graph: Anaemia in young females with dispositions to very delayed menstruation or suppression of it. Menstrual discharge is offensive. Feels always cold.

Sepia: Puffed. Flabby persons; dirty-brown, blotched skin. Very much sensitive to cold air. Not inclined to do any work.

ANGINA PECTORIS, BREAST-PANG

Therapeutics Leading Indications

Acon: Greal anxiety with fear of death. Full, strong and throbbing pulse, or feeble, thread-like pulse. Suffocative constriction of chest, so distressing that he sweats from agony. Pain in region of heart, going down left arm: *Esp.* indicated in strong, plethoric subjects.

Arsen: Anxious restlessness with weakness. Can only breathe very gently with chest stooping forwards. Least motions makes him lose his breath.

Cact: *Feeling of constriction at heart, as if an iron band were preventing its normal motion. Acute pain in region of heart with difficulty in breathing.

Spig: Exceedingly sharp pain worse from any motion. Palpitation so violent that it is visible and audible. In complication with organic diseases of heart.

***

Amyl-M: Violent beatings of heart; intense throbbing of heart and carotids. Flushing of face. (Mother tincture put on a little cotton placed in a vial to be inhaled.)

Lach: Choking, constriction or rising in throat, with organic diseases of heart. *Very much distressed after a short sleep.

Rhus-t: Painful stiffness all over. Violent palpitation when sitting quietly. Pain extends to left arm.

Phyt: Pain goes to the right arm or right side.

ANUS, AFFECTIONS OF

Fissure of Anus: It consists of an abrasion or ulcer near anus. This is generally very sore. Therapeutic hints are given below.

Condurango: Fissure at anus with terrible pains when bowels are moved.

Nit-ac: Even soft stool is expelled with much difficulty and pain; as if rectum would be torn. *Sharp, splinter-like pricking pains during and burning after stool.

Sepia: When shooting pains run up into abdomen associated with bleeding piles.

Thuja: Painful to touch, often with warts, *esp.* in syphilitic subjects. Fissures deep and may contain pus.

***

Caust: Pain worse and bleeding when walking. Fissure burns like fire.

Silica: Great pain for half an hour after stool, lasting several hours.

Fistula in Ano: It is a pipe-like sore with a narrow opening, penetrating into the tissues about the anus and into the rectum itself. It is often based on tubercular diathesis. Surgical operation often leads to tuberculosis of the lungs.

Berb-v: Fistula in ano. Passing of stool with violent burning in anus, as if surrounding parts were sore with bilious symptoms. When fistula in ano has closed up after it has been operated upon, and shooting, twinging pains and other sufferings (short cough, chest complaints) appear in their turn (Calc-p., Silicia.).

Caust: Pain of excoriation and moisture in anus.

Thuja: Fistula in ano with general symptoms of the remedy. Pains in anus worse from motion.

Phos: Ulceration of rectum with discharge of pus and blood,

Nit-ac: Fistula and ulceration of anus; pricking pains. Prolepses ANI Recti: Inversion and falling down of lower part of abdomen. Often associated with piles is adult. This is prolapses of anus.

Nux-v: With constipation; in persons of sedentary habits, frequently useful in children.

Ruta: Immediately on attempting at stool; sometimes with stool. When caused by overstraining a stool. Frequent unsuccessful urging to stool.

APOPLEXY

Popularly called a 'stroke', a 'fit'. Sudden loss of consciousness, total or partial, with greater or less disturbance of pulse and respiration, arising from congestion to head and hemorrhage into the substance of the brain.

Acon: Sudden attacks of congestion in young and robust persons. Full, rapid, strong pulse. Redness of face throbbing carotids, paralysis of tongue. Great difficulty in swallowing.

Arnic: Due to fall or any mechanical injury. Paralysis limbs, *esp.* of left side. Head hot, rest of body cool. Stupor with involuntary passing of stool and urine. Slight fever. Bar-c: of aged persons and drunkards. Paralysis of limb or right side or general paralysis (in patients who are old). Disturbed consciousness, acts childish.

Bell: Red. Bloated face, difficulty in swallowing, throbbing carotids, attack being sudden. Paralysis of limbs, right side Loss of sight, smell and speech. Mouth drawn to one side involuntary urination.

Glon: In persons who are prone to apoplexy, who suddenly well-known streets seem strange. To combat chronic disposition to apoplexy. When attacks recur frequently, (Kafka).

Lach: Paralysis of left side. Mouth drawn to one side (Bell.). *Cannot bear anything to touch his neck. Entire inability to swallow. After abuse of liquors (Nax-v., Bar-c.).

Nux-v: Preceded by nausea and urging to vomit paralysis of lower jaw (mostly, of lower extremities, which are cold and without sensation).

Opium: Most important in all bad cases. Lies unconscious; eyes half-opened; respiration laboured; snoring and rattling. Face dark red and swollen. Sometimes titanic rigidity of body. Sinking of lower jar. Continual grasping at head. (N.N. When the patient is stupid and drowsy, there is often lack of reaction and indicated remedies fail to respond. Optimum rouses the vital forces from their lethargic condition and paves the way to a cure. Lilienthal says: "Give Apis or Nux-v., where Opium fails." This means that when comatose condition or dizziness of the mind fails to yield to Opium, Apis or Nux-v. comes to the rescue.)

Hyos: Fall down suddenly with a scream. Red face, mobility to swallow, dropped jaw. Involuntary passing body. (For all these clear-cut symptoms, if Hyos., fails, Arnica often helps.)

Anac: Loss of memory; weakness and confusion of sight. General paralysis.

Caust: Paralysis of single parts. Gradually appearing paralysis. Tendency to make mistakes when speaking. Inability to select the proper words. Paralysis of extremities.

Cup-m: Paralysis of tongue; speech imperfect and stammering. Mental functions remain undisturbed.

Plumb: Comprehension difficult; loss of memory, cannot recall words to express himself. Progressive loco-motor ataxia. Constipated, cannot strain at stool. Trembling of tongue when it is put out.

APPENDICITIS

Inflammation and swelling in the ileocecal region, just under the abdominal wall, being movable upon the swollen part which may be soft or hard. May be due to foreign bodies or to infection by bacteria.

Therapeutics Leading Indications

Bell: Great pain in the ileocecal region, cannot bear in least touch, not even the pressure of the cover and, above all the least jar. Is constrained to lie motionless on back.

Bryon: Abdomen very sensitive and sore; have swelling; stitching, tearing pains worse from least motion constipation.

Colch: Has worked wonders in many hands seven times. Its action is incredibly quick. It must be watches to be believed. Affected part is extremely sensitive to touch and pressure. Great distension of abdomen. Griping, tearing, cutting, stitching pains. Motion excites vomiting; aggravates pain. Even least vibrations render pain unbearable. Extra prostration. Cold feeling in abdomen. Aversion to food loathing even the sight or still more, the smell of it.

Hepar: Deep, circumscribed swelling in the ileocecal region. Lies on back, with right knee drawn up an easiest position. Great sensitiveness to slightest touch. Cold sweat on head.

Lach: Rapid onset of the disease. Abdomen high sensitive to touch. Burning pains. Can only lie on bed with the knee drawn up. When turning to left, sensation of rolling of ball in abdomen, particularly after the formation of pus. *Feels worse after sleep.

Rhus: Hard painful swelling of nearly the entire right side of abdomen. Pain worse from sitting or whose stretching the right leg. Impossibility of lying on left side. Better when lying on back with right leg drawn up.

Thuja. In sycotic persons. Sweats only in covered parts; or all over except head, sweats when he sleep sweating stops when he wakes. Relief of pain by flexing the legs; aggravation from stretching them Relief of pain from very light rubbing of the parts. Pain relieved by wrapping up.

Mer-s: Painful, hard, hot, red swelling in ileocecal region; painful to touch. Sweats without relief. Tendency to suppuration.

Plumb: Large, hard swelling in the aforesaid region; painful to touch and least motion, or when sneezing or coughing. The abdomen is drawn in, cheeks retracted, sunken. Pain radiates to other parts of body or in all directions.

ASPHYXIA-APPARENT DEATH (GAS POISONING)

Therapeutics Leading Indications

Ant-t: Asphyxia from drowning (Lach). From foreign bodies in larynx and trachea (Silic). From mucus in bronchi. From impending, paralysis of the lungs (Pneumonia). All these conditions are characterized by drowsiness and comatose conditions.

Ant-t: In such a state of apparent death, has either pale face or dark, red face, and may have blue lips. Asphyxia in the newborn; infants at birth pale, breathless, gasping; rattling of mucus in throat.

China: From loss of blood. Also in newborn babies, after loss of blood by the mother. From Poisoning by Fumes of Burning Charcoal: Carboneum sulphuratum is an important remedy for asphyxia from alcohol and also from coal gas. It has cold sweats and sudden attacks of general trembling.

From Other Causes: After a fell, with shooting and jerking, try Hyper. After a blow or fall, have recourse Arnica. Opium is indicated in asphyxia from hanging or from a stroke of lightning.

ARTHRITIS-GOUT

Painful inflammation of usually the smaller joints occurring at longer or shorter intervals, consequent upon the accumulation of an excess of uric acid in the blood which is too much for the kidneys to eliminate. As per result thereof, it deposits itself into the joints or other localities of the body, producing painful inflammation.

Therapeutics Leading Indications

Abrot: Joints stiff, swollen, with pricking sensation, wrists and ankle-joints painful and inflamed. When gout is suppressed and heart is attacked.

Ammon-phos: Constitutional gout with nodes out concretions of sodium urate in the joints.

Arnic: Joints sore and tender; *constant fear of being touched.

Benz-ac: Gout engrafted on a gonorrheal or syphilitic constitution; urine has *very strong urinous odour, smells strong like that of a horse, urine being dark brown. Gouty conceretous. Nodes in Joints. Swelling and pain of right knee. Gout going from left to right; from below upward pains change place incessantly, but are constant about heart.

Berb-v: Gouty and rheumatic states are associated with liver and kidney disturbance, with violent sticking, cutting pain extending from kidney into bladder and urethra. Old gouty constitutions.

Caust: Gout and rheumatic inflammation with contraction and stiffness of joints. Must move them constantly, but motion does not relieve. Tendency to paralytic weakness.

Colch: A great remedy to gout, *esp.* in robust vigorous constitution. Extremely acute pain, making the patient scream when touched. Pains go from left to right. Small joints particularly affected.

Ledum: Gout, whether acute or chronic; begins in lower limbs and ascends; pain and swelling proceed upwards and heart becomes affected. Pains worse from worth and *better from cold applications.

Lyco: Chronic gout with Calcarea deposit in joints; uric acid deposit in urine. When headache is worse, gout is better and *vice versa.* Presence of copious quantity of red sand in urine leads to elimination of headache and gouty pain.

Apis: Oedema of affected parts; very tender to touch; relief from cold water.

Bryon: Aggravation from slight motion and touch.

Kali-bi: Pain of fingers, alternating with gastric symptoms; periodical wandering pains.

Lith-c: Border of foot and soles as if gouty; pain in ankles and bones of feet; excess of uric acid deposit in urine.

Mang: Pain in joints shifting from one joins to another or crosswise; worse at night; worse in cold, damp weather.

Rhodo: Pains excited or aggravated by cold damp, windy weather.

ASTHMA

Therapeutics Leading Indication

Ant-t: Asthma of children and old people. Great rattling of mucus in chest with inability to expectorate: When the patient coughs, it seems there is a large collection of mucus in the bronchi, but nothing comes up. Relief after expectoration.

Arsen: A valuable remedy in asthma, whether acute or chronic. Great oppression of breathing, must spring out of bed at night, *esp.* after midnight: unable to lie down for fear of suffocation; *must sit up bent forward. Feeling as if dust is being inhaled. *Great anxiety and restlessness. Asthma from suppressed itch.

Hepar: Anxious, wheezing, moist breathing; worse in dry, cold air; better in damp. Wheezing or purring sound in chest.

Ipec: Spasmodic form of asthma with violent contraction of throat and chest. Rattling or wheezing in bronchial tubes, yet nothing is expectorated. In stout persons of lax fiber, either adult or child.

Kali-bi: Expectoration of tough, tenacious mucus. Asthma worse from 3 to 4 O'clock in morning. Asthma which is liable to return in winter or in summer who are chilly.

Kali-c: Asthma and cough worse from 3 to 4 O'clock morning has to sit bent forward to breathe during attack, resting head on knees. Asthma relived by rocking.

Lach: The patient arouses from sleep with asthma attack. *Cannot bear anything around throat and chest. Finish coughs up a large quantity of watery phlegm with relief worse after a meal; after talking; from moving arms; for touching throat. Better sitting bent forward.

Spong: Asthma worse after sleep or sleeps into an aggravating suffocative attacks of breathing without any mucus respiration loud, wheezing, whistling, sawing, anxious, when at full moon.

Bar.c: Asthma of children with enlarged tonsils and swelling of glands.

Bell: With sensation of dust in lungs. Better bending head back.

Brom: Asthma of sailors as soon as they go ashore. Gasping and suffering for breath with wheezing and rattling in larynx; accumulation of too much of phlegm in larynx. Sensation as if air passages were full of smoke.

Bryon: Worse from least exertion or talking. Stitches in chest, worse during inspiration, when coughing or during motion.

Carb-v: Of old, debilitated people, who look as if dying during attack; blue and cold skin; *desire to be fanned. Chronic, once or twice monthly.

Cup-m: Attacks come on suddenly and after some hours cease suddenly. Face gets blue; threatened convulsions.

Ferr-m: Worse after midnight, driving out of bed; better by walking slowly about, and talking and uncovering the chest.

Nux-v: Asthma from gastric disturbance; worse in morning from cold air, after eating or exercise; belching relieves.

Senega: Low potencies in watery solution are often of great benefit. This is Nash's testimonial. Great soreness of walls of chest. Great accumulation of mucus in larynx and trachea, which is difficult to expel. Symptoms may be most violent during repose.

Spong: Asthma depending upon tuberculosis. Dry asthma; the patient rouses up generally after midnight with fear of suffocation and death; wheezing respiration; sputa cannot be raised, must be swallowed, swallowing ameliorates. Rawness in chest.

BEDSORES

Therapeutics Leading Indications

Anth: Of a malignant type with gangrene and terrible burning. Sores horribly offensive. (When aresn. Though indicated has failed.)

Arnic: Bathe the parts with water to which a few drops of arnica mother tincture has been added. Also administer it internally in the 30th or 200th potency. Odour of sore is offensive. Great soreness of parts.

Arsen: Burning relieved by heat; offensive.

Carb.v: Parts bluish; burning; putridity.

Crotal: Of a malignant type; from degraded state of blood; prostration of vital force; fetid odour.

Lach: Edges are black.

Secale: Dry gangrene; skin withered; aggravation from external heat.

Hippoz: Sores have livid appearance and have no disposition to heal; putridity.

Sulph: Gangrenous sore; burning; gnawing pain.

Sulph-ac: Putridity; rapid spreading; gangrenous tendency; weak and exhausted, weakness being out of all proportion to the disease.

BITES AND STINGS

Therapeutics Leading Indications

Stings of Insects

Amm-c: has the reputation of counteracting the effects of the stings of insects. It is also of great use in many cases of snake-bites as would be evident from the following symptoms: oozing of dark, thin blood, coldness, stupor, cyanosis, prostration etc.

Ledum: Is the supreme remedy in stings of beast. While I was at Gaya (Bihar), a boy while plucking guavas. Feel down from tree. The injury consist of more than dozen of stings.

Ledum: is also called for in mosquito and rat bites.

Arnica: Hemal writes, "The water of arnica is most excellent application to mosquito bites, bee stings etc." Hering says: "For stings of insects give Aconite and some 6 hours later Arnica. If not better, the next dose is Nat-mur."

Apis: It is supposed to be a splendid remedy in stings of insects, *esp*. bee-stings, but I have no experience with it. It has burning, stinging pains and much swelling the affected parts.

Arsen: After stings of poisonous insects, if Ammo, Ledum, and Apis fail to do any good within 10 minute, try Arsenic and then, Anthracinum *esp.* when the affected parts get inflated (oedematous) and burn like fire.

Lachesis: In cases of stings of poisonous insects. When even Arsen, fails try Lach., *esp.* when fainting takes place and the swelling looks bluish.

Bites of Dogs

For bites of dogs, whether rabid or not, administer Bell. In watery solution in oft-repeated doses for two days. Gradually increasing the interval from half an hour to two hours. After that if anything not towards would happen, administer Lach. Or Lyssin. For headache from bites of dogs, whether rabid or not, give Lyssin. Clarks writes, "The effects from bites of non-rabid dogs have been removed by this nosoed."

In a case of dog-bite (whether the dog was rabid or not), (I cannot definitely say), I was called upon to undertake the treatment. The patient was badly bitten and was having fever. I effected a speedy cure by administering a few dose of Arsenic 30, having recourse to no other remedy.

Bites of Snakes

The bite of a venomous snake is our next subject. More homeopathy can do much better than any other system of treatment. Tightly tie a rope or ribbon around the bitten limb, just two or three inches above the part. Above this ligature tie a few more, one being above the other and two or three inches apart. Then the poison will have to be sucked out of the wound with all possible force by the patient himself or any other attendant provided the former or the latter has no sore in the mouth, lips, gums, or the tongue. Then the wound should be incised and the parts washed by Permanganate of potash for half an hour of more. After this process, the ligatures may be unfastened. During this procedure the patient should not be allowed to fall asleep.

After having recourse to tight bandaging as per directions already hinted at and after sucking out the poison from the wound, if possible, apply heat at a distance, say one-fifth of an inch or so from the wound by means of a glowing charcoal or a burning cigar held directly over the wound and at the same time covering the surrounding parts of the wound with oil, or it that is not a hand with saliva. Heat is to be applied for at least one hour on until the patient begins to shudder and to stretch, or until the effect of the poison wears off. After the wound have been thus treated, rub the wound with common salt. And the same time give the patient a little salt-water to drink from time to time. Should dangerous symptoms make their appearance, let the patient drink one or two tea-spoonful of alcohol (wine, brandy, whisky etc.) every three or four minutes until improvement sets in, and resume giving brandy as soon as symptoms reappear.

This is the method described and recommended by Hering. Now give a dose of Arsenic 30 every half an hour according to requirement on the following indications. Rapid prostration; shooting pains growing worse and proceeding towards heart: vomiting, fainting, giddiness, wounds become bluish, checkered like marble, swollen, if Arsen. fails, have recourse to Bell. 30 (or 3x) on the indications: Sleepy but cannot sleep; face red, hot, bloated great dryness of throat; pupils immovable and dilated sweat on covered parts; mouth open, constant chewing etc.

After ligating the parts as per directions already gives and sucking out the poison, one of the best method to deal with a case of snake-bile (when the snake is poisonous is to poison the patient in the dynamic plane by administrating Lachesis in 30 potency, Naza and Crotolus. Administering the following snake-poisons in potencies one after the other in oft-repeated doses. I would peeler the 30 potency of Lachesis (Surukuku snake), Naja (Cobra Cortiles — Rattle-snake), and even Elapse coral (Brazilian coral snake). The result will be that the patient would be saved, no matter how, in an overwhelming majority of cases, even including those cases have been declared as absolutely hopeless. This is a secret that leads to success. This is my own method, although it is more or less empiric. For want of space at my disposal, I have eschewed elaboration.

Before administering these snake-drugs, give the patient Arnica 3X, 30, even 200 in repeated doses. Arnica often have the way to a cure. Mother-tincture of Echinacea Angustifolia in 10-drop doses frequently repeated has the reputation as a remedy in snake-bite. The medicine is equally good in stings of poisonous insects.

Senega (Mother-tincture) enjous the reputation of relieving the symptoms of snake-venom. It also antidotes bites of poisonous animal or an animal when it is in a state of rage.

BOILS

A small hard inflamed tumor when becomes pointed sometimes after its formations and finally suppurates.

Therapeutics Leading Indications

Acon: Boil highly inflamed; fever with dry, hot skin.

Arnic: Crops of small boils, which are very painful and sore to touch.

Bell: The inflamed part looks red, sometimes very and (Firey red or of erysipelatous appearance); burning, throbbing. Dryness of mouth and tongue.

Berb: Suppuration (Hepar, Merc-s.). *The pains radiate from the part affected.

Hepar: The boil is very painful to touch; throbbing pain. Here it hastens suppuration. Administer a dose of Hepar 200.

If there is sticking or pricking pain in the boil. Hepar is sharply indicated.

Merc-s: When pus is coming out and is scanty after pus has formed (never to the given before the formation of pus). Pain is throbbing. Burning, stinging. Bloody pus.

Sulph: Boils coming in crops in various parts of the body. A single boil or a crop of boil is succeeded by another as soon as the first or the first crop is healed (Tuber.). When there is a strong predisposition to and frequent relapse of the disease.

BONE DISEASES

Therapeutics Leading Indications

Angus: Caries and painful ulcers which attack the long bones and perforate them even to the marrow Necrosis of lower jaw.

Asaf: Caries of nasal bones. Ulcers affecting bones discharge of thin, ichorous pus; ulcers are intolerably sensitive to touch around edges; easy bleeding; pus thin ichorous and putrid.

Aur-met: Ulcers attacking bones. Caries *esp.* of cranial bones and bones about nose and palate, with tearing, boring and burning stitches and offensive discharge. Nightly aggravation of pain. Caries in consequence of syphilis, *esp.* after abuse of mercury.

Calc-f: Bony growths with or without caries; hard rough, corrugated evaluations on bones; osseous tumors ulceration and suppuration of bones.

Fluor-ac: Has eroding effect on bones, *esp.* long bones. Facilitates expulsion of necroses parts, and thereafter, heals the affected bones. Discharge of carried thin, acrid, offensive. Even pus is excoriating. Dental fistula; discharge bloody, selfish, of disagreable taste.

Ruta: In bone injuries. Formation of deposits is periosteum, in bones. Effect of bone injuries often come insidiously. It cares hardened spots and nodular growth left after bruises.

Silicia: Bones very sensitive and tender to touch, bending and caries of bones.

Kali-bi: Swelling of bones after syphilis: Nit-ac. Noddes hard and painful: Phyt.

BRAIN-FAG

Therapeutics Leading Indications

Kali-br: Bad results from overtaxing brain. Brain numb, confused; content drowsiness.

Nux-v: With gastric symptoms; cannot use mind two or three hours after a meal, worse towards morning.

Pic-ac: Brain-fag from study and mental exertion. Mental prostration after reading a little; after writing a little. Least study causes burning along spine and other symptoms, such as, lameness, soreness, heaviness, diarrhoea etc. Slight mental exertion brings on headache.

Phos-ac: From over-work, loss of vital fluids, *esp.* seminal, by sexual excesses. Least mental exertion causes heaviness in head and also in limbs. Trembles, legs and back weak. Indifferent to the affairs of life. Profuse urination at night.

Mag.c: Exhausted nerves; lassitude, *esp.* in feet. Unrefreshing sleep; more tired on rising.

Zinc: From over study; from too much of mental labour; from night-watching. When wear and tear of tissues are faster than the process of replenishment and there is a fagged condition. Fidgety feet.

BRONCHITIS, ACUTE

Therapeutics Leading Indications

Acon: Short, dry cough, worse evening, night with tickling in throat.

Ant-t: On coughing. It seems as if much would be expectorated, but nothing comes up. Coarse rattling of mucus. *esp.* useful in children and old people.

Bell: Sweat on covered parts. Dry, barking spasmodic cough in paroxysms. Child cries when coughing; starts and jumps in sleep.

Bryon: *Dry cough which hits head and chest, holds them with hands.

Eup-perf: Soreness in trachea and bronchi; Lace flushed, tearful eyes. Patient supports chest while coughing, to relieve pain and soreness (Bryon., Nat-s). Inability to lieon left side.

Gels: Dry cough with soreness of chest and fluent coryza; hoarseness with dryness of throat.

Hepar: Dry spasmodic barking cough with a wheezing breathing. Sometimes loose, rattling and choking cough. Cough worse early morning hours. (Often called for after Acon., Ant-t., Ipec., Sponge.). Bronchitis after repelled eruptions.

Hyos: Dry, spasmodic cough worse when lying down relieved by sitting up (Dros.); worse at night.

Rumex: Teasing periodical dry cough, *Decidedly worse in cool air; pain in chest. *Cough ceases when head is covered with bed clothes. *Cough ceases when mouth covered up to exclude cold air.

BRONCHITIS, CHRONIC

Therapeutics Leading Indications

Amm-c: Chronic bronchitis; of the aged: copious accumulation of mucus in lungs; dilation of bronchial tubes. "Numerous coarse rattles, and yet he experiences no necessity to clear his throat." Coughs continually without any expectoration or a little expectoration with great difficulty. Aggravation in winter and from 3 to 4 a.m. Great weakness.

Calc-c: Sputa yellow, lumpy, sweetish, sometimes putrid; when thrown into water, a lump is seen shooting to the bottom with a mucus trail behind, like a falling star. (Fellger).

Carb-v: *Esp.* indicated in old neglected cases, and where the constitution is exhausted and in aged. People, expectoration profuse, sometimes purulent, putrid. Cold knees even in bed.

Dros: Cough spasmodic, deep sounding, worse after midnight. Tightness of chest when coughing.

Hepar: See the previous article.

Hydra: *Thick, yellow, tenacious expectoration. Tongue shows imprint of teeth. In old people with debility. Loss of appetite; loathing of food. Feels suffocated when lying on left side.

Kali-bi: Expectoration of tenacious, stringy mucus, which can be drawn out into long strings. Desire for acid drinks. Early morning cough.

Kali-c: Scanty, tenacious expectoration, difficulty to dislodge, must be swallowed. Cough worse at about 3 a.m. pain in lower chest have, exhausted look; face bloated; sensitive to cold.

Lyco: Rattling of mucus in chest; oppressed breathing; pain as from a bruise in chest.

Nit-ac: Pain as from excoriation in chest; putrid small from mouth; whistling inspiration; shortness of breath. Chronic winter cough. Broken down constitution.

Silic: Expectoration of pus, which when thrown into water, falls to the bottom and spreads like a heavy sediment (Felloer). Expectoration thick, Yellow, Lumpy; purulent. Cough worse from cold and better from warm drinks.

Stan: Profuse greenish expectoration of an offensive, sweetish taste. Sensation of great weakness in chest after expectoration or talking.

Sulph: Rattling of mucus in chest. Fated expectoration of a greenish-yellow colour, like pus, and of a salt or sweetish taste. In cases where seemingly indicated remedies fail to act.

BURNS

Applications of moderate heat to the affected parts in the case of superficial burns and scalds is often sufficient. (Let likes be cured by likes.)

In superficial as well as in deep burns, one of the best remedies and an easily procurable one is soap. Make a thick solution by mixing soap with warm water, spread it over a piece of linen and apply it to the burnt or scalded surface. The dressing should be renewed once in twenty-four hours. If blisters have formed, they should be punctured with a needle. For superficial burns and scalds, external application of alcohol is of great service.

Therapeutics Leading Indications

Cantharis: But for superficial burns and scalds there is no remedy like our cantharis. I have derived equally good results from the mother tincture as well as the 30th potency for external application. Apply a linen soaked in mother tincture or the 30th potency of Cantharis. The effect will be magically instantaneous, and no after effect would ensue. Cantharis prevents the formation of blisters.

Causticum: It is very useful for after-effects of burns and scalds; in old sores originating in burns. Internal administration of a dose or two of the 30th potency is often quite sufficient to ward off the ailments. For scalded tongue the action of Causticum is amazing, as I have often observed.

Crotal: When burns threaten erysipelas or gangrene, give this remedy, which is also of use when hectic fever is developed.

Carb-ac: When affected parts ulcerate and the discharge is ichorous, offensive, it is of great service.

Secale: In gangrene after burns when the part looks blue and is cold, administer Scale. And when in such part there is lack of sensation, Scale is the remedy. For burns from nettles, use Caust.

CANCER

A malignant tumor terminating is a fatal ulcer. An affection of constitutional origin. Such tumor is not necessarily painful and may or may not be associated with anaemia and emaciation.

Therapeutics Leading Indications

Arsen: Cutting, burning pains like fire; relieved by heat; pains *worse after midnight. Cancer of stomach with similar symptoms, relief being from hot drinks. (When Arsen. fails, Ars-iod. May be useful. If Ars-iod. Fails, try An thracinum.). Spongy excrescence on thumb.

Brom: Cancer of breast; stitching pain from breast to armpit, cannot bear pressure, Swelling and in duration of neck glands, which enlarge slowly.

Carb-an: *Esp.* cancer of breast. Cancerous ulcers surrounded by hardened tissues which are bluish or blue, red; burning; offensive, acrid discharge. Cancer of uterus; neck of uterus indurate; thin, offensive discharge; burning pain.

Conium: Ulceration based on cancerous diathesis. Cancerous ulcer on lip (from the pressure of the pipe). Cancer of stomach. Cancerous swelling of stony hardness. Sharp, stitching pains; usually painless.

Condurango: Cancer of tongue. Cancerous tumors or ulcers with painful crack. Breast Cancer; nipple so retread as to be invisible.

Hydras: Of great fame in cancer. Cancers are hard, adherent; skin mottled, puckered. Cancer of breast, with pain like knives thrust into parts. Cancer of stomach; vomits everything except water and milk; emaciation. Cancer of tongue, of liver.

Kali-car: Cancerous ulceration of right side of tongue. "Cancer of tongue, edges indurate, raised and knotty, speech difficult and indistinct, cannot masticate on account of pain."

Kreos: Cancerous ulceration of the neck of uterus, with hardness, burning, sensitiveness, discharge being bloody, putrid, profuse, corrosive. Vitality reduced. Cancer of stomach; painful, hard place on left side.

Lapis alb: Of much repute in uterine cancer. Cancer of breast. With burning, shooting, stinging pains. When ulceration has not set in and is associated with scrofulosia (Glands not hard but to a certain extent elastic and pliable). Discharge horribly offensive. Lapis came into play when Arsen through indicated had failed.

Phos: Cancer of stomach: particularly when it is about to pass into the stage of ulceration; vomiting of food as soon as swallowed or cold water as soon as it gets warm in stomach; vomiting of a sour, foul-smelling fluid.

Secale: Inflammation and cancer of stomach; vomiting of food with great debility; burning. Cancer and gangrene of uterus; offensive discharge from uterus causing her vomit.

CARBUNCLE

An extensive flattened boil, very little raised above the level of skin but very deep-seated. Attended with burning, smarting pain. Usually associated with fever and other constitutional disturbances and generally accompanies diabetes and albuminuria. Surgical interference does no good. Homoeopathy has won laurels in combating this virulent type of disorder.

Therapeutics Leading Indications

Anth: Carbuncles with *terrible burning pains; discharge of chorus offensive pus. All openings run into one; copious discharge of pus. Poisoning of blood by absorption of pus; typhoid symptoms. Stinging.

Apis: Burning, stinging; erysipelatous (Anth, Tarant.).

Carb-ac: Offensive discharge; great prostration, paleness of surface and cold sweat; low fever.

Crotal: Degraded state of blood; discharge scanty, tardy and of dark fluid; dark, scanty urine; prostration of vital force.

Hepar: If given early in high potency, it sometimes aborts the disease; later it promotes suppuration. Edges of ulcer burn and sting; discharge corroding, little pimples surround the ulceration.

Kreos: Great soreness; discharge hot, burning, acrid, offensive; bluish; easily bleeding.

Lach: Bluish or of purplish appearance; *great sensitiveness to slightest touch; when suppuration is tardy, Carbuncles which slough and are very offensive (Anth.). Systemic weakness.

Nit-ac: Putrid decomposition with tendency to bleeding; excessive debility with copious night-sweats. *Prickling, stinging, as if from splinters running through.

Rhus-t: Intense pain and dark red swelling in the beginning; great restlessness; pain to a certain extent relieved by moving about.

Silic: "During the process of ulceration it clears the wound of its decaying masses and promotes healthy granulations." Particularly carbuncle between shoulder and nape of neck. When the part is intractable and hard. *Esp.* indicated in the supportive stage, Fistulous opening with offensive discharge. It removes in duration after carbuncle.

CATARACT

Opacity in crystalline lens of the eyes, or its causing partial or total blindness.

Therapeutics Leading Indications

Calc-c: Spots and opacity of cornea. Stony cataract is gouty subjects. Constitutional symptoms of the remedy.

Calc-f: An effective remedy in cataract. I cured a case with the 200th potency. Stony cataract in arthritis subjects. Senile cataract.

Colch: Rapidly forming capsular cataract; soft. From general perversion of health.

Nat-m: This is common salt, which has produced opacity of crystalline lens in dogs and so Nat-m. is supposed to cure cataract.

Silic: From suppression of foot-sweat; from defective nutrition and after inflammation of eyes.

Sulph: After skin affections, *esp.* suppressed itch (Psor.) left eye affected. Cortical cataract. Dim vision. Dr. Jhar says that he accomplished most with Sulphur. Allowing a dose to act a long time. After exhaustion of the action of Sulphur, he generally resorted to Calc-c. and then to Lycopodium.

Chel: Gray cataract. Aching in eyeballs on moving them.

Euph: Light seems obscure and violating. Capsular opacity. Clarks prescribes Euph. Mother tincture ten drops to an ounce of water, three times a day.

Jaborandi: One part of the mother tincture of the remedy diluted with five parts of water may be used externally. This sort of medications may cure many cases of cataract. Blurred vision for distant objects.

Tell: Chalky looking white mass on anterior surface.

Note: Senega has the reputation of promoting absorption of cataract. Carbon-an. and Secale sometimes play their role in cataract affecting old people. The third remedy in such cases is Cineraria maritima. Clarks writes that it has been used with a good deal of success in cases of cataract as an external application. "Drop into the affected eye, four or five times a day, one drop of Succus Cincrar. Marl. and keep it up for some months." (Clarks). He further writes: "Traumatic cataract and corneal opacities, as well as senile cataract, have been removed in this way. I have seen no report of cures by internal use of the remedy alone, not in some cases it was given internally as well as externally. Generally, the patients have received specific homoeopathic treatment at the same time." Needless to add that in any case of Cataract, constitutional homoeopathic treatment is also essential.

CHOLERA

An attack is often recognized by marked weakness following one or two evacuations. Violent purging and vomiting attended with griping pain in stomach, cramps in legs, prostration, cold extremities etc. At times vomiting and purging may be entirely absent. This is called 'Dry Cholera.'

Therapeutics Leading Indications

Acon: When symptoms set in suddenly and with great intensity. Loose stool with cutting pain in abdomen (Acon. Inor 3x given on this indication often aborts the disease). Great anxious restlessness and fear of death. *Predicts the wave of Death. Unquenchable thirst for large quantities of cold water.

Arsen: Anxiety; mental restlessness. Fear of death. Drink often but little at a time. Watery stool, profuse and offensive, smelling like carrion or of putrid odour. Violent burning in stomach and bowels. Worse after vomiting. Vomiting immediately after eating or drinking, particularly anything cold. Worse after midnight. Pulse scarcely perceptible. Surface of body as cold as ice but internally the patient complains of intense burning heat. Still wants to the warmly covered (opposite to Secale). Skin covered with cold clammy sweat. Profound prostration. (Rice-water stool does not indicate Arsenic).

Camph: Cholera sets is violently without vomiting and purging, but with other serious symptoms, such as, sudden sinking of all strength, icy coldness of body (But cannot be covered like Secale), groaning with squeaky or husky voice etc. Cramps in calves. Face pale, icy cold. Distorted suppression of urine. Disappearing of pulse. (Gradually glow of the body and perspiration indicate its good action on noticing which the medicine should be discontinued.)

Carb-v: When an attack begins with hemorrhage. From bowels, or when associated with great flatulence. Cyanosis (bluish countenance). *Desire to be fanned, air hunger. Coldness of legs to the knees. Cold breath, cold tongue. Copious cold sweat. Vital forces nearly exhausted. Pulse intermittent, thready. Distension of the abdomen. Stool very offensive.

Colch: Nausea, vomiting, purging of rice-water stool. Violent distension of abdomen. Great prostration, Hippocratic face, cramps, coldness, and last but not least, rice-water stool constitute a remarkable combination in Cholera, Burning or icy coldness in stomach. Profuse cold sweat. Loathes even the sight of food. Cholera in autumn. Remember that Colchicum is primarily indicated by the actualness and violence of an attack. (A case was declared as hopeless by allopath. At the last stage a homoeopath administered Cuprum met. On the indication of violent cramps of calves. Cuprum added fuel to the fire. On the indications (i) rice-water stool, (ii) Cramps, (iii) violence of the disease, (iv) nausea and vomiting, and (v) influence of change of weather, it bring autumn, when days were hot and nights were cold, "I hastened to my dispensary close by (without further study of the case by the bed-side) and immediately sent six doses of Cloch. 30, to be given every three minutes. The action was as speedy as it was marvelous.

The storm lost all its fury as if be some freaks of nature. Later on, three doses of Ricinus 30 has been given for completing the cure." Bhanja.

Cup-m: Spasm or cramp is the most prominent symptom. Violent cramps in different parts of the body, particularly of muscles of calves and thinghs. Cramps of muscles of throat, preventing speech. The fingers and toes are inclined to be bent inwards (unlike Secale). Cuprum cramps are at times so violent that the affected muscles are drawn up into knots. Cramps begin from the extremities (fingers and toes) and spread over whole with gurgling sound. Great coldness and blueness of surface, with prolonged cold sweat and great sinking of strength. Urine scanty or suppressed. Nothing characteristic about stool.

Kali-p: Kali-p. 12x trit. (biochemic) is almost a special in cholera. Stools like rice-water; very offensive. Crave for ice-cold water. Abdomen distended.

China: In the beginning. Undigested food particles appear in stool. Distension of abdomen, temporally ran relieved by belching.

Lach: *Esp.* indicated in cases where the patient without being much affected by one or two evacuating thereafter all of a sudden stagers and falls down as it struck by lightning and passes stools and vomits unconsciously, stools very offensive.

Phos-ac: Before vomiting has set in. Discharge of stool painless copious, odorless. Discharge not weakening. Great rumbling. Stool generally whitish, watery Cholera morbus.

Podo: Profuse watery stool, gushing out like water fire an bung-hole, as if through a syringe; frequent urging and evacuations; stool yellow. Offensive. Violent cramps of feet, calves, and thighs. Rumbling in abdomen.

Puls: When no two stools are alike thirstlessness.

CHOLERA INFANTUM

Therapeutics Leading Indications

Anth: In severe form of the disease. Stool light yellow or greenish.

Vomiting is curdled milk or milk is thrown up just as it was swallowed. After vomiting exhaustion and sleep (due to debility). Spurns with clenched thumbs; *eyes turned down; cold limbs.

Arsen: Great restlessness; extreme prostration; skin dry and shrivelle; stool offensive. Generally begin after midnight (Sulph.). Vomiting excited by least quantity of water taken.

Cal-c: Child smells sour (Mag-c., Rheum). *Esp.* in fat, children; legs cold, damp. Stools chalk-like; undigested.

Zinc: When caused by fright or suppressed eruptions; great depression of spirits. Worse during rest. Fidgety feet, constant motion of feet while in bed. Choriec movements better from exercise.

COLIC

Pain in abdomen of a purely neuralgic character. Without any pathological changes in the intestines. Flatulent colic is characterized by distension of abdomen; gastric colic is due to over-eating; lead colic originates in handling lead as in the case of compositors of press who have to manipulate lead types.

China: Flatulent colic, *esp.* after eating and at night. Distension of abdomen with sensation as if packed full, not in the least relieved by eructation. With shivering. Violent pains about navel relieved by bending double. After exhausting illness.

Cup-m: Violent pains as if a knife were penetrating through navel to back, with fearful distressing screams. Pain better from pressure, but not relieved by heat. Cramps in abdomen. Abdomen is drawn in (Plumb.).

Lyco: Colic in lower part of abdomen with suspended respiration; fullness and distension of abdomen. Cutting pains across abdomen from right to left. Belching without relief.

Nux-v: Flatulent colic with difficulty in breathing (due to upward pressure of accumulated flatus). Colic due to sudden stoppage of flow from piles. Lead colic.

Plumb: Horrible griping pain in abdomen which radiates to all directions (Dios.), generally following the course of nerves.

CONVULSIONS

Therapeutics Leading Indications

Bell: Flushed face, red eyes; fever; hot head; cold feet; during teething. Drowsiness after spasms. Child plump and large-headed.

Calc-c: Often required after Bell. When that remedy has no lasting effect. Delayed dentition with characteristic sweat on head and open fontanels.

Cham: Stiffness and bending backwards. Legs move up and down gasping and reaching with the hands; mouth drawn from side to side; eyes staring; hot sweat about face and head. One side of face red, the other pale; very irritable; must be carried all the time to be quieted.

Cina: Worm complaints; picking and boring at nose; face pale. Becomes suddenly stiff, followed by trembling of whole body. Gurgling noise during spasm, as if water were poured out of a bottle from throat down to abdomen.

Cup-m: With clenched fingers and blue face; with screaming out: boring the head into pillow, spasms begin in fingers and toes and spread into whole body. Caused by dentition; by repercussed eruptions, or failure of eruptions to come out.

Hyos: Sudden starting and twitching of muscles; one arm twitches, then the other. Trembling and foam at mouth. Face deep red. Caused by fright or worm.

Ignat: Spasm returns at the same hour everyday. Single parts or single muscles twitch (particularly those about eyelids or mouth). here and there convulsed.

Opium: Caused by fright; in infant when its wet-nurse has become frightened or angry; begins with loud screams; foam at mouth; trembling of limbs; eyes half open; face dark red and hot. Hot sweat on body. Deep snoring sleep after attack.

Stram: Violent convulsions, with violent distortions and ever heamorrhage. Twitching of facial muscles or of Single or isolated groups of muscles *esp.* of upper part of body Dribbling of glairy saliva from mouth.

Lach: When occurring during sleep; Trembling of tongue; cold feet before attack; with screaming; sleep after attack.

CORNS ON SOLE OF FEET

Thickening or hardening of skin, chiefly on toes or soles of feet. As a palliative treatment, soak the affected part in hot water and when softened, pare down the corn and bathe it with a lotion of Arnica (30 drops of the mother tincture to a wine-glassful of water).

Ant-c: Corns on soles of feet which are very tender. Callous excrescences under nail of great toe. Ant-c. corn is often inflamed.

Petrol: Corns have burning and rawness.

Ran-b: Very similar to petrol, which has bruised soreness in corns as well as burning. (Both Thuja and Sang. Have burning corns.)

Ignat: Corns painful as if sore.

Bovis: With violent shooting pain in corns.

Nat-m: Corns in patients who crave for salt and salty things.

Dois: Corns feel as if jumping and darting.

CORUPLENCY (GREAT OBESITY)

Therapeutics Leading Indications

Ant-c: Often useful in great obesity, particularly in children and young people. The patient feels exhausted in warm weather; perspires a good deal from slightest exertion.

Calc-a: Suited to fat persons, *esp.* fat women approaching climax is, all of them bring very sensitive to cold weather (they feel some sort of inward coldness) and their liver and spleen being somewhat enlarged.

Caps: Fat, indolent; clumsy in motion.

Graph: Comes into play in women, inclined to obesity, who suffer from habitual constipation, with a history of delayed menstruation: feels always cold indoors or out; easily chilled and easily overheated.

Lac-d: A reputed medicine for obesity and fatty degeneration. Particularly indicated in very fat women who feel completely exhausted, whether they do anything or not.

Phyto: Has the power to absorb abnormal tissues and new growths (such as tumors etc.) and hence its applicability to obesity.

While all the aforesaid remedies may be used in potencies (30, 200 or even higher according to sharpness of indications). Phyt. It reputed to be efficacious in the form of mother tincture, two or three drops being a dose.

CORYZA

Therapeutics Leading Indications

Aconite: When caused by exposure to dry, cold air. Attended with chilliness, which may be followed by fever with thirst. Checked coryza with headache, better in open air. Fluent corzya, frequent sneezing and dropping of clear, hot water, two or three doses of Aconite 30 every one hour is almost always sufficient. If there is fever, never repeat a dose as soon as perspiration sets in.

Bryonia: Is often called for after Acon. At time after Nux vom. It has great dryness of the mucous membrane of the nose. Lips parched and dry. Headache worse from motion. Discharge thick and yellowish. When such discharge becomes suddenly suppressed resulting is throbbing headache.

Allium cepa: Profuse, watery, corrosive discharge from nose; worse in evening and in a room and better in open air. Discharge ceases in open air but returns on coming into a warm room. Lachrymation profuse and bland (it does not excoriate the cheeks); burning in eyes. Allium cepa, even when indicated, is at times a treacherous remedy, as the disease force thus driven from nose tends to spend itself on the chest. Here phosphorus often saves the situation. (Phosphorus indications are: Tightness across the chest; great weight on chest. Just a single dose of the 30th potency is required. It may do harm if repeated.).

Ammon-carb: Nose is stopped up at night; wakes up gasping for breath; long-continued crazy.

Dulcamara: Dry coryza with stoppage of nose; excited in cold change of weather and in damp weather.

Gelsemium: Summer colds with early morning sneezing. Liability to catch cold at any change in the weather. Nasal discharge excoriating; edges of nostrils red and sore. Chilliness with desire to hung the fire. Languid, wants to lie down.

Pulsatilla: "Ripe" cold, discharge being yellow or rather yellowish green, thick and bland (no excoriating effect).

Sabadilla: Spasmodic sneezing, with running nose. Copious watery, nasal discharge. Coryza with severe frontal pains and redness, and watering of eyes. (*See* influenza.).

COUGH

A symptom of various diseases ranging from most simple affections like cold in head to most fatal affection like phthisis.

Therapeutics Leading Indication

Acon: Short, dry cough; arising from tickling in throat: caused by exposure to dry, cold air; worse evening, night. May be with fever.

Ant-t: Cough sounds loose; coarse rattling of mucus is heard in chest, but little or no phlegm comes up. *Esp.* useful in children and old people.

Bell: Dry, tickling teasing cough; from tickling in throat as from dust. Spasmodic cough worse at night, waking from sleep. Cough often compels patient to sit up, but sitting up causes no relief (opposite to Hyos.).

Bryon: Cough hurt distant part of the body, such as, head and chest, holds them with hands. Cough dry, spasmodic, with gagging and vomiting. Worse from motion. Pain and soreness in chest, must press hands upon chest when coughing to relieve pain. Stitches in chest (Kali-c., Squilla).

Caust: Dry cough; cannot cough deep enough to raise mucus for relief; what little is about to be expectorated must be swallowed.

Drinking cold water relieves cough. During cough involuntary spurting of urine (Nat-m., Phos., Puls., Silicia) hoarseness worse morning; soreness and rawness of trachea, but not of chest.

Cina: Spasmodic cough with gagging. Cough so violent as is bring tears and pain in the sternum. Worm symptoms.

Dros: Spasmodic cough ending in gagging, retching and vomiting, prolonged periodical fits of choking cough; cough compels patient to hold the sides. Worse evening, night, after midnight.

Hepar: Dry cough, worse in morning. Croupy, choking cough with loose rattling phlegm. Cough excited by slightest exposure to fresh air.

Ipec: Cough with fine rattling or rather wheezing in bronchial tubes, from large accumulation of mucus; as a rule phlegm does not yield to coughing, threatens suffocation.

Kali-bi: Cough with expectoration of *tough stringy mucus which hangs down in a ropy string (Hydras.).

Nux-v: Dry, fatiguing cough from titillation in throat; worse early morning; after eating or drinking. Pain in head or abdomen when coughing (Bryon., Caps., Lyco.).

Puls: Cough dry at night (loose during day) going off when sitting up in bed (Hyos.) and reappearing when lying down. Expectoration yellowish, green; bitter.

Rumex: Dry. Incessant, violent, fatiguing cough cause by tickling in throat pit; worse evening and night after lying on left side, touching or pressing throat-pit.

Spong: *Cough is dry in all respects. Excited by dryness in throat; caused by dry, cold weather; sounding viciously dry (barking, crowing and even sawing); everything is perfectly tight and dry. (This is how I have depicted the drug-picture in my work "Master key to Homoeopathic Malaria Medical."). Nash.

Stan: In phthisical subjects. Great soreness in chest after every cough; sensation of great weakness and emptiness in chest. Expectoration yellow or green; *sweat; seltish.

CRAMPS

Therapeutic Hints

In abdomen: In cholera; Hell., Iris. In cholera morbus; dios., Podo. Of these Dios. Has sharp cramping pain in stomach followed by belching or large quantities of tasteless wind relieving distress at stomach. In various parts of abdomen: Gels. During pregnancy: Gels, Hyos. In Navel Region—Dios. Has griping, cramping pain rumbling to bowels; wind colic.

In Arms: In cholera morbus: Jatroph. Writer's cramps; Anac., Caust., Gels: of lesser importance, Nux-v., Ruta, Secale, Steph., Zinc. Cramp—like pain: Cina, Kreos.

Calves: Obliged to get out of bed and walk for relief: Rhust-t. In cholera: Ant-t., Camph., Colch., Cup-m, Jatroph, Kali-p., Mag-p., Sulph., Ver-a. With watery diarrhoea: Mag-p. In dysentery: Colch., Merc-c. Muscles become knotted: Jatroph. In morning in bed: Caust., Sulph. At night: Mag-c., Nux-p., Sepia, Sulph. Cramps in calves and soles, *esp.* at night, must stretch feet out: Nux-v. When walking: Sulph. Sepia is our important remedy when no cause is traceable. Sepia has also cramps in things when walking. Nit-ac. Has violent cramp *esp.* at night and towards morning, as well as on walking after having been seated.

In Feet: As if about to be cramped: Dios. Mostly in daytime: Sepia. Sepia has stiffness is heels and joints in feet, as from contraction. In soles: Caust., Colch., Sulph. In soles at night: Carb-v., Nit-ac. In Asiatic Cholera, soles particularly affected at night : Sulph. In soles, during pregnancy: Calc-c.

In Fingers: As if about to be cramped: Dios. In cholera: Colch., Cup-m., Ver-a. Drawing out of shape: Carb-v. (which has also cramp, like contraction of hands.). Distressing during pregnancy: cup-m. In thumb: Nat-m. In writers, piano, organ or violin players: Mag-p, stan.

In Muscles: Now here, now there: Caust. In broken-down constitution: in zymotic or malignant diseases: crotal.

In Thighs: Agar., Hyas., Sepia, Sulph.

In Toes: Caust., Crotal., Cup-m., Dios. In pregnancy Calc-c., Cup-m.

Nux-v: Has cramps in several parts of the body. Rhus-t-has cramps during day, *esp*. when sitting still. Refer to the article on Colic.

DANDRUFF

Therapeutics Leading Indications

Alumin: Dryness of hair. Itching in scalp with profuse desquamation. Want of vital heat.

A m m-m: Itching dandruff; hair falls out. Obesity. Itching of skin, generally evening.

Calc-c: Dandruff; painful. Sensibility in root of hair.

Graph: Abundant desquamation of scalp. Scalp itches very much. Falling out of háir. Hair turns gray.

Nat-m: When scalp is greatly sensitive. Abundam falling of hair (as soon as it is touched).

DENTITION

During the period of dentition children are liable to attacks of fever, diarrhoea, convulsion etc. Dr. Herring says that during this period constant dribbling and looseness of the bowels may be looked upon a salutary, as these have the effect of preventing congestion of the brain or lungs. Any condition which is however, particularly abnormal should be combated homeopathically.

Therapeutics Leading Indication

Acon: Child cries and whines; constant gnawing at its fingers or fists, or something else. Watery diarrhoeas. Characteristic fever.

Bell: Moans and groans a food deal; starts suddenly from sleep as it frightened; face and eyes red, head hot. Gums swollen and inflamed (*See* the article on Convulsions.).

Calc-c: Difficult and delayed dentition with characteristic head sweat during sleep; open fontanel's. Abdomen Large and hard; cold damp feet. Stools like lumps of chalk or are thin and whitish. Sour vomiting of large curds. (*See* the article on Convulsions.)

Calc-p: Stool green and slimy or thin greenish; great flatulence; refuses to nurse or nurses all the time.

Cham: Starting and jumping from sleep; very irritable, quiet only when carried: stool green, slimy mucus, of like chopped eggs and spinach, smelling like rotten eggs. Gums red and tender; one cheek red and hot, the other pale and cold.

Kreos: Very painful dentition. Gums bluish red, soft; spongy. Great restlessness, wants to be constantly in motion, screaming all night.

Merc-s: Gums are livid, and discolored; copious salivation; profuse sweat at night.

Podo: Rolling of head during dentition: restless sleep with half-closed eyes; moaning and whining during sleep. Profuse watery stool gushing out like water as if through a syring stool is quite offensive.

Phyt: Wants to continually bite teeth or gums together or to bite continually on something hard.

DIABETES MELLITUS

True diabetes characterized by frequent and immoderate discharge of urine containing sugar or glucose, attended with excessive thirst, rave nor hunger or loss of appetite at a later stage, progressive wasting of the body and increased debility. Food containing starch and sugar should be avoided. The following articles of food are allowed: Cabbages, cucumbers, cauliflowers, tomatoes, onions, greens, lemons, acid fruits, meat, fish, milk, butter and ghee.

Therapeutics Leading Indications

Arg-m: Frequent desire to make water, with profuse emission, *esp*. at night. Appetite greatly increased, feels hungry after eating a full meal. Great dryness of mouth; emaciation; great weakness. Particularly indicated when scrotum, ankles and feet are oedematously swollen.

Arsen: Great hunger and unquenchable, agonizing thirst. Emaciation and great weakness. Excessive urination. Useful in diabetes with dropsy.

Kreos: Frequent and urgent want to make water; copious pale urine; thirsty. Putrid odor from mouth. Painful weariness in all limbs.

Lactic-ac: Urine contains sugar; great thirst; large quantities of sugar are passed frequently; skin rough and dry; there may be constant nausea, or nausea on awaking; better by eating. Obstinate constipation; stool hard and black, slight exertion causes exhaustion; debility. Associated with rheumatic pains in joints.

Phos-ac: Urine looks like milk or lime water, or like jelly after standing. Profuse watery urine containing much sugar. Profuse, watery urine which forms a white cloud at once. Indifferent to the affairs of life. Great debility; emaciation.

Plumb: A medicine of repute. More frequent and more copious emission of urine. Weariness and dislike to conversation and labor. Violent thirst *esp.* for cold water. Violent hunger even after a meal. Sweetish or offensive taste. Emaciation gradually develops. Diminution of sight. Loss of sexual desire and impotence.

Thuja: It has sugar in urine and indicated by the general symptoms, Thuja works orders. Notice if the patient has dropsically bloated face.

DIARRHOEA

Therapeutics Leading Indications

Acon: Useful at the very onset of acute diarrhoea. Stool watery; green like chopped spinach, slimy, Cutting pain before and during stool. Useful in so-called hill-diarrhoea.

Arg-n: Stool green, slimy, shreddy, like chopped spinach a flakes. Turns green after remaining on diaper. Stool is expelled with much spluttering, i.e., much noisy flatus. Provoked by eating sugar-candy.

Arsen: Stool yellow, watery; dark or black; profuse and brownish yellow; excoriates anus. Offensive, smelling like carrion. Burning in anus and rectum during and after stool. Vomiting immediately after eating or drinking. Great exhaustion after stool.

Calc-c: Stool whitish; watery. Smelling like rotten eggs; sour-smelling profuse sweat on head in sleeping.

Carb-v: Involuntary; putrid; and is cadaver smelling; flatus putrid or inodorous. Worse from 4 to 6 p.m.

Cham: Stool hot; green watery; yellowish watery, chopped eggs and spinach; smelling like rotten eggs. Soreness of anus. Colic during and before stools. Peevishness.

China: Stool yellow, watery, undigested; involuntary putrid, painless. Distension of abdomen (whole), temporally relieved by belching, great weakness. Worse at night after a meal.

Ipec: Stool: grass green, mucus; fermented, dark. All black, looking like molasses. Nausea and colic before during stool. Clean tongue.

Nit-ac: Chronic diarrhoea. Stool is putrid, and offensive; green, slimy with tenesmus. In the children syphilitic parents.

Nux-v: When due to alcoholic drinks. High living, medicines or prolonged drugging. Pain and tenesmus case stool. Worse early morning.

Podo: Profuse stool, gushing out as if through a syringe offensive; worse morning, hot weather. Rumbling in abdomen.

Puls: *No two stools alike, stools constantly changing in colour and character. After fruits, ice-cream, after rich fat food. Worse at night. Irresistible desire for cool, fresh air Bitter taste in mouth. Thirstlessness.

Sulph: Early morning diarrhoea driving the patient out of bed; as if bowels were too weak to retain the contents. Stool may contain undigested food; Smell of stool clings to patient for a long time, as it lies had soiled himself. Excoriation, about anus.

Thuja: Diarrhoea daily in morning; daily after breakfast forcibly expelled with much noisy flatus. Gurgling like water from a bung-hole. *Esp*. in chronic diarrhoea.

DIPHTHERIA

A dreadful, infectious disease characterized by fever. Prostration and formation of white, yellowish white or grayish while deposits of various thickness, most frequently in throat, which is inflamed, attended in some cases with swelling of glands of the neck.

Therapeutics Leading Indications

Apis: Diphtheria progresses insidiously with a little pain but, much inflammation, or from the very beginning great prostration with high fever and drowsiness. At first, throat appears coated with glossy red varnish; membrane assumes a dirty-grayish colour, Stinging and burning pain in the affected parts. Oedema of throat; uvula odematous and elongated. (Merc-cy. Follows well.)

Arsen: In some respects Arsen. In similar to Apis, but is required in later stages and in severe cases. Membrane dry-looking and wrinkled; gangrenous, very strong, offensive odour. A dynamic fever; great anguish and restlessness; great and increasing prostration.

Brom: Diphtheria begins in larynx and extends up wards; chest pains run upward. Sometimes the direction of extension is reverse. Diphtheria begins in throat and invades larynx and then extends down to the respiratory organs associated with great prostration with may be described as "deathly weakness".

Ignat: Dr. Raue goes so far as to say that he found it acting well in all cases, although he could not make out any particular indication on which to prescribe. It is, however, apt to be indicated by a sensation as of a lump in throat which is not felt while swallowing anything but felt after it. This lump sensation is attended with soreness which is worse between the acts of deglutition.

Kali-bi: Discharges whether from nose or throat are tough and stringy; the disease spreads upwards into nostrils and downward into larynx and trachea; hoarse, croupy cough: offensive smell form mouth.

Lach: Diphtheria begins on left side and extends to right; membrane more marked on left side. Dark purple appearance of the swollen parts. *Liquids cause more difficulty in swallowing than solids; throat pain worse from empty swallowing or swallowing saliva. Symptoms *worse from hot drinks; *after sleep. Air hunger; must have open air for relief. Pain in throat runs up into ears. Great prostration in the very beginning. Great sensitiveness of throat from external touch.

Bapt: Creat prostration, lies in a stupor; discharge from mouth and nose putrid, horribly offensive. Can only swallow liquids.

Nit-ac: Nasal diphtheria; discharge from nose watery and very offensive, excoriating every part is touches (like Arum, after which Nit-ac. Follows well); putrid odour from mouth; *sticking, picking pain as from splinters.

DYSENTERY

Characterized by frequent urging for stool with pain in abdomen, great tenesmus (straining), scanty mucous stool, which may be bloody, and feverishness.

Therapeutics Leading Indications

Arsen: Stool dark of blackish fluid, mixed with blood of putrid, foul smell; during stool tenesmus and burning in rectum.

Bell: Stool thin, green, mucous; bloody mucus with great tenesmus, during and after stool. Tenesmus so served as to cause shuddering. "it is often the only remedy required for severe cases of infantile dysentery." (J.K. Bell).

Bryon: During hot summer, From taking cold drink when overheated. Pain and stool provoked by motion even by turning in bed. And, for this reason, wants to keep very still.

Canth: White or pale radish mucous stool, like scraping from intestines, with streaks of Blood (Carb.ac., Coloc,), with tenesmus of rectum and even bladder.

Caps: Tenacious mucus, streaked with black blood. Violent tenesumus in rectum and bladder at the same time. After dysenteric stools, craves ice-cold water, which, however causes shuddering.

Colch: Stool Jelly-like mucus; white or bloody mucus having a shreddy appearance, looking as if the lining membrane of the bowels were scraped off. In all violent cases, remember this friend of ours, no matter if the symptoms would tally or not. Also in sutumnal dysentery. In there is violent tenesmus followed by spasms or constriction of the mouth of the anus.

Coloc: It is another friend of ours whom we often fail to remember or recognize. Stool slimy and bloody looking like scrapings of the intestines. Before stool cutting colic and great urging; during stool cutting colic and great urging; and great tenesmus; temporary relief after stool. Dysentery with colicky pains, often relieved by pressure in the beginning but, later on, pressure aggravates pain. Aggravation of symptoms from least motion is in my opinion highly characteristic. Dysenteric stools renewed each time by the least food or drink (Remember that in dysentery with great tenesmus Merc-s. is complementary to Coloc.).

Crotal: In rural areas, many dysentery cases of septic origin are met with caused by drinking foul water or food. These cases I have successfully combated by Cortal 200 (two doses having been given in each case). There may be dark, fluid blood in stool associated with great prostration.

Kali-bi: Bloody, Jelly-like stools (with morning aggravation). After Canth. Has removed stools like scrapings of the intestines, they will often become jelly-like, sometimes stringy. Here Kali-bi. Often comes into play, which has painful urging, tenesmus and gnawing pain in stomach during stool.

Nux-v: Stool bloody, mucous, frequent, scanty and very unsatisfactory, with sensation as if more has remained behind. But it is almost exclusively indicated by; *marked relief of pain and tensemus for a short time after stool. Morning aggravation.

Aloe: Stools bloody or transparent lumps of jelly, with griping stomach, usually relieved after stool. Much flatus loud gurgling in bowels.

Arnic: Stool slimy. Bloody, and offensive. Great urging and tenesmus during stool, relief after stool. Long intervals between stools.

Carb-v: Mostly in advanced stages. Frequent involuntary stool (with flatus of putrid, cadaverous small). Great prostration and symptoms of collapse.

Ipec: Stool dark, almost black, looking like frothy molasses, with violent colic and tenesums. Much nausea and vomiting.

DYSMENORRHOEA (PAINFUL PERIODS)

Painful menstruation, often attended with scanty menstrual flow. In membranous dysmenorrhoeal, shreds of membrane of the uterus are discharged with the flow.

Therapeutics Leading Indications

Apis: Violent labour-like bearing down pain; stinging pain in ovaries; inflammation of right ovary.

Bell: Pain precedes flow; sensation as if everything would come out through vulva; relief from sitting erects; pains come on suddenly and cease suddenly.

Cham: Flow of dark, clotted blood with tearing in thigh; severe labour-like pain in uterus; great irritability. Hot sweat about head; one cheek red, the other pale.

Coloc: With violent paroxysmal pain, better from hard pressure and heat, with great nausea and vomiting and cold feet (these symptoms may manifest themselves several days before menses).

Conium: During flow, sensation of bearing down and dragging in thigh, or painful cramp in abdomen. Breasts flabby. Nervous debility. Scanty menses.

Mag-p: Crimpy neuralgic pain, severe, intermittent , preceding flow; may continue during flow; better from heat, worse from motion. Flow may be dark, fibrinous, neuralgic dysmenorrhoea.

Puls: Scanty menstrual flow comes by fits and starts; colicky pain with tossing about and crying; pain doubling her up: Chilliness; thirstlessness. Feels smothered in a closed room. In spite of chilliness, wants to be in open air.

Secale: Foul-Smelling, blackish discharge. Pain of an expulsive character in uterus. Skin cold, but cannot bear to be covered.

Sepia: Scanty discharge: crimpy colic with sensation of bearing down as though the contents would issue through vulva, must cross her legs to prevent protrusion of parts.

Cup-m: Violent cramps in abdomen extending into the chest. Convulsion of limbs. Piercing shrieks. Flow more profuse during night than during day (Amm-e., Zinc.) with dragging pain, better from pressure on abdomen and stooping.

Phyt. With erosion and ulceration of the neck of uterus; breasts are hard and painful. Complicated with rheumatism.

Potency question: The lower dilutions of the following remedies are generally used. Gels. 1x, 3x (also 30, from which I havc got good results). Viburnum 3x. Seneria 1x or 3x. Mag-p. 6x (Also 30, which I always have recourse to with desired effect). A few doses of the indicated remedy may be used a day or two before the attack comes on.

DYSPEPSIA, INDIGESTION

Therapeutics Leading Indications

Ant-c: From over-loading the stomach, Stomach weak, digestion easily disturbed. Belching with taste of what has been eaten. *Thickly coated white tongue. Loathing nausea. Distention and distress about the abdomen. Disorder of recent date.

Arsen: Loss of appetite; loathing of food. Least food or drink causes distress and pain, or immediately excites vomiting, or stool or both together. Vomits all kinds and grades of substances. Irritable stomach of drunkards.

Bryon: In hot weather or from drinking cold water when overheated. Everything tastes bitter (Pulls.). Food distresses the patient as soon as taken. Pressure in stomach after eating as from a stone (That means that food lies in stomach like a heavy load).

Calc-c: Chronic dyspepsia. Pressure as of a weight in stomach. Loss of appetite, but when he began to eat, he relished it. Sour vomiting and ravenous hunger in the morning. Cannot bear anything tight around waist. Craving for eggs for indigestible things, such as chalk, charcoal etc. Milk disagrees. "Disgust and repugnance for meat and to warm or cooked food, desire for cold victuals."

Carb-v: Digestion slow and imperfect. Aversion to meat and fat things, to milk which causes flatulence. The most innocent food distresses. Sensation as if stomach and abdomen would burst when eating or drinking. Distension of stomach temporarily relieved by belching. Stomach feels full and tense with flatulence, with tendency to diarrhoeal. Flatulence is most troublesome in upper part of abdomen. This flatulence presses upwards. Eructation's sour.

China: Slow digestion, food remains long in stomach. Abdomen feels full and tight, not in least relieved by belching. Continual sensation of satiety. Aggravation after a meal at night and distension after eating a little.

Hepar: The stomach is easily disordered, despite strict dietary and utmost care. Craving for acid food and drinks and condiments and wine. Empty sinking feeling at stomach. Strong and comfortable feeling after a meal. Chronic dispepisa. Chronic diarrhoeal.

Lyco: A feeling of satiety alternating with a feeling of vigorous appetite. But this appetite is quickly satisfied as soon as the patient begins to eat. Distress in stomach fell immediately after eating (*N.B.* Puls., Nux-v., and Anac have distress in stomach about two hours after eating. Irresistible desire for sleep after eating. Constant sense of fermentation going on in the abdomen. Heartburn. Sour eructation, acid in stomach. Great desire for sweets (Arg-n.).

Nux-v: *Esp.* when cause by mental over work. Distress in stomach, coming on an hour or two after meal, not after the digestion is complete, there is not distress. Frequent ineffectual urging to stool. Heartburn. Sour eructation. The patient is very irritable.

DENGUE (BREAKBONE FEVER)

It is an acute, infectious, endemic and epidemic tropical disease. Occasionally, it is attended with eruptions. The disease is characterized by fever, severe pain in the bones and muscles. There may be inflammation, swelling and pain in the joints. One feels as if bones are broken. As if the long bones of the legs were detached from the ligaments.

Dengue is a Spanish word. Suggesting prudery. This name is significantly applicable to this disease by reason of the face that in Dengue, there is stiffness of the patient's neck and shoulders, portraying an affected reserved state or overdone strictness of manners. If I am called upon to christen this disease by a Sanskrit name, I would propose the designation, pangne, in view of its paralyzing effect on muscles to a degree that is most annoying and at times exasperatingly painful.

The period of incubation is from three to four days. The attack comes on suddenly; Fever is very often high, temperature rising to a maximum limit of 106 degree F. It is caused by a virus transmitted by mosquitoes, especially by Ades aegypti.

After fever has subsided, residual ailments of various kinds continue for even months. Unless checked by proper medication.

In my experience there was an epidemic in Calcutta nearly forty years ago. Later on, dengue in this city was almost conspicuous by its absence. The year 1964 is marked by very wide-spread invasion of this disease in Calcutta and in many parts of the Province. Although it is seldom fatal and complications are raze, it is still a most abominably lingering disease, convalescence being in many cases notoriously slow.

It has been very recently declared by our Government that no prophylactic remedy of this disease has so for been discovered. The question is whether any prophylactic remedy for any other disease has so for been found out for instance, whether vaccination has been fruitful or whether it is deleterious in its effects is a question in which even opinions of eminent physicians of the Allopathic system of treatment vary to an alarming extent.

Therapeutics Leading Indications

Arsen: Great debility; great thirst, but drinks little at a time, although often, bone pains. Constant drowsiness, with strong and frequent yawning. Chilliness without thirst. Rapid failure of strength, and sensation of weakness as if from want of food. Inability to walk; the patient is obliged to remain lying down. Hugs the fire and likes warm wrapping. Anxiety; restlessness.

Bapt: As soon as the patient feels malaise (Bodily discomfort, before the development of the disease). Give the patient 3 doses (I drop dose) of the remedy every one hour and two more doses thereafter every four hours or so. By adopting this procedure the disease may be either aborted or its virulence counteracted to a great extent, paving the way to a cure by some other remedy or remedial according to indications. General muscular soreness. Too lifeless to move. Great langour, want to lie down. Weak and tremulous. Breath, stool, urine, sweat—all offensive.

Bryon: Joints red, swollen and hot; pains worse on least motion. Knees stiff and painful. Rheumatic pains in limbs, with tension; worse form motion; better from pressure. Refer to the article on Fever (simple).

Colch: Great weakness with sensation of lameness in limbs. Pains in joints are extremely acute and unbearable. Joints stiff, feverish. Internal coldness. Urine dark, scanty or suppressed. Aching in lumbar region. Backache, better from rest and pressure.

Gels: Feels sore and bruised all over the body. Giddy, confused; muscles refuse to obey the will. Fever, thirst less, full, dusky-red face, chilliness. Desirous of lying still.

Eup-perf: Great soreness and aching of whole body as if in bone. Deep hard aching, as if in bones. Intense aching in limbs and back as if bones were broken, (3x in watery solution to be administered every 20 minutes: 8 doses. Later on, 30th may be used in infrequent doses.).

Rhus-tox: Whole body painful. Soreness and bruised feeling fluffiness of affected joints.

Bell: Sudden onset of the disease. Great burning of mucous membrane. Failing of strength, paralytic weakness. Aching in the eyes and the sockets. Painful and difficult deglutition. Painful stiffness and cramp-like pains in the sacral regions and in the back. Stiffness in hip, after sitting for some time, with difficulty in getting up. Tottering walk, the legs refuse their service. Fever, cold limbs with hot head. Sweat on covered parts only.

China: Weakness and want of stability in the coxolemoral joints, the knees, and the ankle-bones, which yield when walking. Sensation of torpor in different parts. Haemorrhagic conditions.

Cal-fluor: In a case of swelling of knees and lack of flexibility in them, preventing the bending thereof, I cured with two doses of the remedy in the 200th potency, administered at an interval of one week. This was the only symptom left behind after the storm was over.

Ferr-met: Stiffness of muscles of neck with pain during movement. Great lassitude and general weakness (almost paralytic). Hemorrhagic conditions. Urine blood-red, contains blood corpuscles.

Hamam: Haematuria; passive congestion of the kidneys; dull pain in renal region.

Ipecac: Pain as from a bruise, in all the bones Haemorrhages from any orifice of the body (blood being bright red). Nausea.

Nux-vom: Immobility of joints. Pain as in bruised it the small of back so violent that he cannot move. Backache; must sit up to turn over in bed.

Secale: Haemorrhage from the bowels; flow of thin black, watery blood, very offensive breath.

EARACHE-OTALGIA

Therapeutics Leading Indications

Bell: It is almost a specific in earache unless the symptoms indicate some other remedy. Shooting pains in ears. Tearing pains is a downward direction. Pains come on suddenly and after a shorter on longer duration, cease suddenly.

Cham: Pressing, stitching pains. Pain in paroxysms (by spells) causing sudden screams. Excessive sensitiveness to pain (becomes furious about it); irritable. Earache with toothache, the latter being relieved by holding cold water in mouth.

Hepar: Great sensitiveness to touch; dread of touch is out of proportion to actual pain. Pain is better by wrapping up and hot application; aggravated by cold application. Hepar is called for after Acon., Bell., Chem., or Puls., when suppuration is imminent.

Merc-s: Inflammation of internal and external ear, with tearing, shooting, drawing and burning pains; pains extend to face and teeth; worse from heat of bed and at night. Sweats without any relief. Particularly when ear is discharging a little. In syphilitic patients.

Puls: Darting, tearing pains and pulsating at night. Pains relieved by cold. Violent pain in ear, as from something forcing outward. Worse in evening and better in open air.

Rhus-t: Earache cause by getting wet.

Sulph: Particularly when the complaint returns frequently and affects the left side. Stitching pain in left ear. "Much itches in ears, changing to pain when attempting to scratch them."

ECZEMA

Therapeutics Leading Indications

Arsen: Dry eruptions with covering like fish-scales, terribly itching and burning being relieved by heat putrid or cadaveric odour.

Anth: Malignant type of eczema with terrible burning pain, relieved by heat and Arsen. Had no effect, oozing eruption.

Calc-c: Moist scabby eruptions with burning and itching. Skin unhealthy; every injury tends to ulceration. Skin excoriated several places.

Clem: Moist, itching terribly; worse washing in cold. Water, from warmth in bed. Eczema worse during increasing moon (when eczema becomes moist), and better during waning moon (when it gets dry). Eczema shows a monthly aggravation at new moon.

Croton: Eczema over whole body with intense itching vesicular or pustule eruption on scrotum and penis with frequent corrosive itching. Croton has itching with is followed by burning pain and the patient cannot bear to scratch very hard as it hurts; a very slight scratch, a mere rub sufficing to allay itching. It has special affinity for skin of the face and of genitals.

Dule: Thick brownish or yellowish scabs, which may form on face, nose, forehead, temples, chins, but *esp*. on cheeks, completely covered with crusts. Aggravation from a cold changes in weather.

Graph: Eruptions cracked. Moist, easily bleeding. Eczema of lids, eruptions moist and fissured. Dry, rough skin that breaks easily and exudes a gluey moisture moist eczema or eruptions behind ears. Moist eczema around mouth and chin. Eczema oozing glutinous fluid which is watery and transparent. Such fluid may be thick, honey-like. Very dry skin; never perspires.

Hepar: Eczema spreading by means of new pimples appearing just behind the original affected parts. Violent itching. Sticking or pricking felt on the parts, which may be painful to touch.

Hydras: Eczema that dries into crusts and burns like fire; worse from warmth, from washing.

Ledum: Gnawing itching, as if caused by lice; burning after having scratched. Red pimply eruptions on face and forehead. Eruptions with burn and sting like the bites of insects (Apis.).

Merc-s: Moist, at times, dry, forms yellow crusts. Burning; stinging; and also ready bleeding.

Nat-m: Eczema: raw, red, inflamed, *esp*. in edges or hair; worse from eating too much salt; worse at sea shore or form ocean voyage.

Peterol: Chronic moist and oozing profusely. Itching while undressing. Feels better in open air.

Rhus-t: With thick crusts; oozing offensive: burning tingling. scratching necessitates greater urging to scratch. Better from warmth in general. Worse in damp or wet weather.

Staph: Eczema of head, ears, face and body; yellow acrid moisture oozes from under crusts.

Sulph: With voluptuous itching (feels so good to scratchy causing soreness and burning after scratching. Dry, scaly unhealthy skin. "Gouty eczema with much oozing."

ENURESIS

Incontinence of urine or inability to restrain urination. Children are apt to suffer from incontinence of urine at night. The first paragraph of this article principally deals with such disorder occurring in children at night during sleep.

Therapeutics Leading Indications

Paragraph-I

Bell: especially indicated in fat, nervous children with fine complexion; involuntary urination during deep sleep, *esp*. after midnight and towards evening. Restless sleep with sudden starting.

Caust: Wetting bed at night during first sleep (Sepia). Involuntary passage of urine when coughing and sneezing.

Cina: Child wets the bed at night, generally during first sleep, with worm symptoms characteristic of the drug. Such as rubbing and picking of nose etc.

Kreos: Urinates when dreaming of the act. Or dreaming of urination in a decent manner, wetting the bed during first sleep (Sepia), from which it is very difficult to weaken the child.

Phos-ac: Children pass a great deal or water in bed (flood the bed) at night. Urgent and irresistible desire to urinate; involuntary urination. All this may be due to self-pollution or sexual excesses in young people.

Puls: Children *esp.* little girls wet the bed at night. Urine discharged by drops when sitting or walking. Involuntary urination during cough; also during sleep at night.

Sepia: Wetting the bed always during the first sleep (Caust., after which it follows well); wets the bed as soon as the child goes to sleep. Urine is very offensive.

Coni: Wetting the bed at night. *Esp.* suited to old men. Frequent emission of urine at night, and sometimes involuntary (cannot be retained). Urine stops suddenly and does not begin to flow again for some moments.

Rhus-t: Incontinence of urine, *esp.*, during report, (at night or when sitting).

EPILEPSY

Attended by loss of consciousness (generally coming on suddenly), convulsive movements of muscles, distortion of the eyes, foaming at mouth etc.

Aura of epilepsy: A sensation of formication, generally lasting for a few minutes before the fit breaks out.

Inhalation of smelling salts during an attack is injurious. Homoeopathic medicines are to be administered when a fit has ceased.

Therapeutics Leading Indications

Absin: Convulsions preceded by nervous tremors; makes grimaces; bloody foam at mouth; consciousness not entirely lost. Terrible hallucinations before attacks.

Agar: Muscular jerking's and twitching, *esp.* of eyes, eyelids and facial muscles. Eyeballs oscillate. Tubercular diathesis.

Bell: Recent case; hot head; cold feet; flushed face; eyes wild, staring, red.

Calc-c: Chronic cases (Silic.), Aura begins in solar plexus and proceeds upwards. Before attack, sensation as of a mouse running up the arm (Sulph.). From suppression of some chronic eruptions (Sulph.). *N.B.* If these symptoms common to sulphur and Calcaria Carb. are present, first try Sulph., and thereafter Cal-c. if Sulph. fails to cure.

Caust: Fit occurs in sleep (Lach.), with involuntary urination. Attacks recur at new moon. Complicated with menstrual irregularities. Aura begins in knees and ascends.

Cup-m: From suppressed eruptions or foot-sweat, or fall or blow on head Aura begins in knees and ascends. Convulsions extremely violent. Worse at night during sleep: worse about new moon.

Hyos: Every muscle in the body twitches, from the eyes to the toes. Without consciousness. Continually touches his genitals.

Kali-br: Caused by sexual abuse or excess in men. Fits occur during or near the menstrual period in women. Occurs at new moon; headache follows it. Slowness of expression and failure of memory.

Lach: Comes *during sleep (Bufo.); from oneness or sexual excess. Aura begins In heart. (The asetrisk is mine. I have cured three cases with Lach. 200 guided by this indication alone. What happens in this: As soon as the patient awakes from sleep, fit comes in.)

Nit-ac: With syphilitic history. Fit occurs after midnight.

Nux-v: Caused by indigestion. *Consciousness with connvulsion. I (had one such case, which yielded to Nux-v. and no other medicine was required.)

Opium: Of drunkards, Screaming before and during spasm. *face dark red; *eyes half-open and turned upwards; stupor. After attack, deep sleep and snoring.

Silica: Chronic cases (after Calc-c.). Attack at night *esp.* about the time of full or new moon. Aura begins in solar plexus and moves upwards. Distortion of eyes. Twitching of lips, lolling of tongue. Before attack, feeling of coldness of the left side of body. After attack, warm sweat.

Staph: From masturbation and excessive sexual indulgence.

Sulph: Chronic cases with psoric taint. From suppressed eruptions. Before attack, sensation of a mouse running up arm or arms. After convulsion, so porous sleep and great exhaustion. History of self-abuse.

EPISTAXIS

Nosebleed, often a symptom of different morbid conditions of the system. If is slight and transient, it requires no treatment, as it is then very often beneficial.

Therapeutics Leading Indications

Acon: In plethoric young people; blood bright red and copious.

Amm-c: *When washing face in cold water, in morning (may be at any time). When aggravated by applying cold water on face. (Dr. Bhanjaee). (I was at my wit's end in a case, in which nearly half a dozen of remedies administered one after the other had failed to do any good.) From time to time, the patient has been washing his face with cold water to clean himself of the discharge. It had been a steady and a long-continued flow of bright red blood. All on a sudden, it struck me that application of water on face caused an increase flow of blood. A dose of Amman-c. 30 less than a minute, he came round.

Arnic: After external injury. When preceded by ting-ling in nose. Blood bright red. From blowing nose. Copious after every excretion (Rhust-t.). From mechanical causes. During whooping cough, typhus etc. Unless contra-indicated and when it is not possible to hit upon any remedy, I always give one or two doses of Arnica 30 with success. The reason is that nosebleed is in itself a keynote of the remedy in my opinion. In the last stage of a horrible case of epistaxis, which baffled the skill of the relational school of medicine, a dose of Arnica 200 cured the patient (a bus-driver in Darjeeling) in less than a minute. The nature of this occupation guided me to the selection of Arnica, when Ipec. though indicated had failed.

Bell: From congestion to head, with red face. Blood bright red and flows freely, drop by drop, even from both nostrils. Worse from motion, noise, bright light.

Bryon: *Vicarious menstruation; epitaxis when menses should appear. Epitaxis particularly at these or four 6 clocks in morning, frequently preceded by sense of fullness in head. When caused in overhanging.

Carb-v: Frequent and long-continued nosebleed *esp.* in morning and afternoon. Great paleness of face before, during and after bleeding. Blood thin and dark in old debilitated persons, in whom the remedy is most useful.

China: Habitual nosebleed, Frequent and long continued, *esp.* morning from six to seven; also with anaemia. *Esp.* indicated when repeated loss of blood had caused weakness, with ringing in ears, pale face.

Ferr-p: Blood bright red, in children. (A case in as anaemic and emaciated women which readily yielded to Ammon-carb., but defied its efficacy after a few hours when it recurred and was characterized by a steady flow of bright red blood was magically cured in my hands by a single dose of Ferr-p. in the 200th potency. (*N.B.* Unless you find a drug homoeopathically called for in a case of nosebleed, with bright red blood, lose no time but try Arnica 30, and then Ferr-p.200, if the former fails. This method is empirical, no doubt, in a sense, but it is calculated to achieve for you success in such an emergency case, where the time factor is most pressing.).

Glon: Nosebleed from sun's heat, face being red and hot; congestion in head which feels large and swollen.

Hamam: Flow passive, venous, long-lasting, blood non-coagulable: feeling of tightness across bridge of nose; fullness of head; bleeding affords great relief.

Ipec: Profuse nosebleed, blood bright red; *heavy, oppressed breathing during; preceded by nausea (rarely met with) . The foregoing asetrisk is mine. The symptom, oppression of breath, having guided me in nearly half a dozen of alarming cases of prescribe Ipec. With laudable success. The action of Ipec. In each case was incredibly quick.

Puls: *Vicarious menstruation (nosebleed from suppressed menstruation.) Bleeding recurs particularly in evening.

Sepia: Violent bleeding of nose during menses. Nose bleeded during pregnancy, child-bed or consequent upon uterine disorders.

Sulph: For persons subject to repeated attacks of nose bleed. Discover the general symptoms of the remedy that correspond with the case. Here refer to Drug pictures in Silhouette.

ERYSIPELAS (LYMPH NODES)

An acute infectious disease "Characterized by a peculiar inflammation of the skin and enlargement of the neighbouring lymph glands, and is accompanied by more or less severe systemic disturbance." The inflammation of the skin is deep seated and is frequently attended by blisters. The affected parts feel stiff, hot and there is burning;, stinging and shooting pains. Erysipelas most frequently attacks the face. So let us deal with such cases first.

Erysipelas of Face

Apis: Eruptions commence about right eye and spread across face of left side. Affected parts quickly become oedematous. Eyelids protrude like sacs of water; *bag-like swelling under eyes. *Soreness and burning, stinging pains. High fever but no thirst. Difficulty in breathing; fidgetiness; suppression of urine.

Bell: *Esp.* affects right side. Surface bright red and smooth, or streaked red (in some cases dark red on account of intensity). Throbbing, High fever.

Canth: Begins in dorstum of nose and spreads to right cheek with formation of large vesicles, which break and discharge an excoriating fluid. Fine stinging and burning pain. Constant desire to urinate, passing but a few drops at a time.

Graph: *Esp.* in chronic cases. Begins on nose (Conth.). Face feels hard and tough; very much distorted. Travels from right to left. Sticky, gummy secretion.

Lach: Most marked on left side. In the beginning face may be bright red, but is soon takes on dark bluish hue. Loquacity, frantic, jumping from one subject to another. Inflammation threatens gangrene.

Rhus-t: Vesicular erysipelas. Face in dusky red. Spreads from left to right. Yellow or bloody serum in vesicles. Itching is very pronounced. Eyelids feel very heavy and stiff. Better from heat. Great restlessness.

Erysipelas in General

The following indication will be guiding in many cases.

Anth: Erysipelas of a malignant type and gangrenous erysipelas. After carbuncle.

Arsen: Pyaemia, Gangrene, Burning and relief from heat. Oedematous swellings. Swelling of the whole body (China.).

Crotal: Called for in most dangerous cases: very feeble pulse; prostration of vital force; cold extremities; hectic fever; pyaemia; dark scanty urine; symptoms worse after sleep. Oedematous swelling during mycosis. After vaccination. *Esp.* adapted to broken-down constitutions.

Strum: Vesicular; violent affections of brain. When erysipelas remains stationary after the administration of Bell. And Rhust-l; Mur-ac. After circumcision: Apis in old people: Lach. Caused by a dissecting wound: Lach. In newborn children, syphilitic or scrofulous: Merc-s.

EYELIDS, AFFECTIONS OR SWELLING OF EYELIDS

Alumin: Chronic blepharitis. Eyelids thickened dry and burning. Agglutination at night and lachrymator during daytime. There may be absence of lachrymation.

Ant-c: Red, inflamed, itching eyelids; slight oozing of skin near external angle of eye. In obstinate cases, the remedy is highly useful, as it has chronic inflammation of lids. canthi raw and cracked.

Apis: Eyelids much swollen, red, *oedemation, *stinging or burning pain, or no pain at all. Relief from cold water.

Arg-n: Thick crusts on lids; canthi red as blood; carancula swollen, standing out like a lump of red flesh.

Arsen: Eyelids oedematous, often completely closing eye. Corrosive tears, making lids and cheeks sore. *Burning relieved by heat.

Bell: Swelling and redness of lids, with heat and burning; great intolerance of light.

Borax: Eyelashes loaded with dry, gummy exudation, sticking together in morning. Granular eyelids.

Euph: Lids red, swollen; lachrymation acrid, profuse and burning. Eyelids itch in daytime and stick together at night: edges covered with scabs or scales and are ulcerated. Sticky mucus on cornea.

Graph: Dry humour in eyelids and in eyelashes; outer canthi mostly affected; they crack and bleed. Chronic blepharitis with characteristic eczema, *esp*. on head and behind ears.

Staph: Margins of lids dry, with hard lumps (Nodules). Inflammation and itching; destruction of hair follicles.

Sulph: Much itching and burning; lid margins thick and granulated; dry crusts in lashes.

Ptosis, Paralysis of Eyelid

Caust: Inclination of close eyes, lids seem heavy; every pain lysis of upper eyelids, *esp*. right side.

Gels: *Great heaviness of eyelids, can hardly open them and keep them open. Ptosis associated with *thick speech (he can hardly speak).

Rhus-t: Heaviness and stiffness of lids, as if paralyzed. Paralytic rigidity of lids, caused by getting wet or working in wet weather; of rheumatic origin.

Alumin: Paralysis of upper lids, *esp*. left. "Very useful when met with in old dry cases of granulation."

Opium: Eyelids hang down as if paralyzed; eye lid half open and are turned upwards.

Sepia: Lids inclined to close as from paralysis; ptosis attended by menstrual irregularity.

Quivering, Twitching of Eyelids

Agar: Generally, the best remedy for twitching eyelids. It has also twitching in eyeballs.

Aurm-t: Quivering of left upper lid, aversion of light.

Croc: Twitching in the upper lid, *esp.* left, worse in the morning.

FACE, PIMPLES ON, ACNES

Bell: Red pimples on temples, in the corners of mouth and on chin. Bright red pimples on face. *Esp.* in chronic persons with red face.

Borax: Pimples on face, nose and lips. Red papules eruptions or, cheeks and around chin.

Caust: Red pimples on face; itching.

Hepar: Pimples of the size of a pea; sensitive to touch.

Kali-br: A very useful remedy for acne. (Use the 30th potency).

Nux-v: From abuse of spirituous liquors.

Phos-ac: Large pimples on face, history of sexual excess in self-abuse.

Puls: In anaemic women with scanty and protracted menstruation.

Sepia: Itching pimples on face; scanty menstruation.

Sulph: When there is burning and itching.

FAINTING

Therapeutics Leading Indication

Coff: Suitable to oversensitive person. When Acon. fails in fainting caused by fright.

Therapeutics Leading Indications

Fluor-ac: Useful in dental (*esp.* at root of teeth) and lachrymal fistula.

Petrol: Has been prescribed by me in lachrymal fistula with great success.

Silic: It a great remedy for fistulous openings in general parts around being often hard, swollen and bluish. When Silica. fails, a dose of Sulph. 30 should be given.

For fistula in gums. Flour-ac. and Slica. are of the importance. When there is tedious suppuration from fistula in gums, use Caust. Other remedies for fistula in gums are : Calc-c., Lyco., Nat-m., Staph., and Sulph.

In lachrymal fistula, when pus in discharged after have been pressed, give Puls. Nit-ac. has lachrymal fistula associated with frequent lachrymator *esp.* when reading with painful sensitiveness of eyes. If there is no pain or any other trouble, except frequent lachrymator, petrol. with in almost all cases cure the malady.

FOREIGN BODIES IN TISSUES ETC.

When dust or any such thing gets into the eyes, never rub them but take it out by introducing small piece of linen which has been previously rolled up. For redness, soreness and inflammation which follow after the removal of dust, coal particles (as from an engine) etc. give Acon. 30 (a dose or two) and thereafter give a dose or two Arnica 30 or 200.

Therapeutics Leading Indications

Silic: It expels foreign bodies embedded in the tissue. In all cases where surgeons are absolutely helpless taking out, say, fish-bones from inside of throat, a single dose of Silic. 30 does the trick in a splendid manner.

In all cases where Silic. has been used to expel foreign bodies (such as needles, splinters etc.) from the tissues. Prescribe a dose of Hepar-sulph. 200 after it in order to aid the healing process.

FRACTURES

In the case of fracture a surgeon's aid is indispensable. At all events, a few doses of Arnica 200 should be administered as it does good in many ways.

After the bone has been set, the compress should be soaked in the mother tincture of Symphytum 30 and then the bandage should be applied. At the same time, Symphytum 30 should be administered internally for a few days, say, three dose per day for the first three days. And later two doses per day for a week or more.

Therapeutics Leading Indications

Symph: Like Ruta it is a sovereign remedy for injuries to bones. Symph. Facilitates union of fractured bones favours production of callus. Lastly, lessens peculiar pricking pains.

Arnic: Most successfully combats profuse suppuration following compound fractures.

Ruta: "It aids in forming callus after fractures, when there is much pain in the injured part." (Lilienthal)

It may be noted that while Symph. And Calc-p. Facilitate union of bones, Arnica and Ruta remove pains associated with fracture. When such pains are not relieved by Arnica, Ruta comes into play, its action being almost never-failing.

Silic: Indicated in malignant and gangrenous inflammation following compound fractures. It expels bone splinters. Also indicated in fistulous opening and offensive discharge, the parts around being hard, swollen and bluish red.

Lach: Gangrenous inflammation of the parts bluish, purplish appearance.

Crotal: Gangrenous conditions; unhealthy suppuration and sepsis.

Anth: Septic conditions with intense burning.

FROSTBITE, CHILBLAIN

Inflammation of the skin on fingers and toes, sometimes ears and nose and other parts of the body due to intense cold in winter, characterized by pain, itching, burning and tingling. Massaging with ice-cold water is of benefit, as it restores circulation and in mild cases affects a cure.

Agar: In the 30 potency (for internal use) worked wonders in my hands, *esp*. in the beginning of an attack. Toes, fingers red, swollen; intense itching; burning; parts feel hot.

Petrol: Particularly when there is a great deal of itching, the parts being moist and sometimes painful. Heel painfully swollen and red. When inflammation sets in with every cold weather.

Phos: When caused by least snap of cold weather, Phos. 30 if administered forthwith, often helps, (Jahr).

Puls: Parts of deep red, bluish or livid. Hue; violent burning and itching; throbbing pains; soles of feet particularly affected. Worse in warm room and *relief from cold applications.

Rhus-t: Burning. Itching pain worse during rest. Itching intolerable at night.

Arsen: Burning relieved by hot applications and tendency to gangrene.

Carb: If Arsen. Is not sufficient give this remedy?

Lach: Parts swollen and look bluish. The affected parts may as well look green, lead-coloured, bluish red or blackish. Gangrenous blisters.

Nat. Mur: Intense burning and tenderness of soles of feet.

Sulph: Thick, red chilblains on fingers. Much itching and burning; worse at night. Skin may crack and there may be much oozing.

External applications: In the beginning chilblains may be rubbed with a liniment of equal parts of strong tincture of Arnica and glycerine. Tamus communis may be applied if the chilblains are very painful and of dark colour. Cantharis lotion is to be applied when the parts are blistered.

GALL-STONE COLIC

Biliary concretion formed in the gall-bladder, or in its ducts are called gall-stone. These concretions may sometimes lie in the gall-bladder for years without giving rise to any trouble. But as these stones pass into the cystic duct, being washed away from the gall-bladder, they produce terrible pain, which goes by the name of "gall-stone colic."

Therapeutics Leading Indications

Bell: The most important remedy during colic according to Dr. Raue. As a matter of fact, it is indicated by the violence of the pain when slight movement or least jar is intolerable.

Barb: Has reputation of quickly and permanently coming gall-stone colic. Twinging, shooting pains/ "Shooting, burning, pressing in the region of gall-bladder; pains come-on spasmodically and are confined to a small-spot; slimy dark urine with heavy sediment, with pains In back and hips. (Lilienthal).

Calc-: Dr. Hughes says that he never failed to relieve gall-stone colic with the remedy. Great chilliness. Darting pain from right to left with profuse sweat. This drug in the 30th or 200th potency may be administered every twenty minutes or so, and if within two or three hours the pain is not relieved some other medicine should be selected.

Chelid: With pain through the lower edge of the right shoulder-blade. Chill with intense pain in region of gall-bladder, and pain form liver shooting towards back and shoulder. Liver tender to touch and pressure. Dirty yellow colour of face. Vomiting. Usually the mother tincture of 2X or 3X potency is used. It has the reputation of expelling gall-stones as well as preventing the formation of the same.

China: Perhaps the best remedy to prevent the recurrence of gall-stone colic and to cure it permanently. The patient should be put on a course of the drug for it few months, gradually using the medicine in infrequent doses. It is principally indicated by the periodic recurrences of colic (although the periods may be unequal and irregular). Indications: Stool undigested; liver is sensitive to touch and pressure; craves delicacies. Dr. Thayer says. "I give usually China 6X six pills twice a day, till ten dose are taken etc. till at length the dose is taken only once a month." And failure in radically curing a case never fell to his lot.

Dios: Cutting pains which changes locality and radiate. A constant pain aggravated at regular intervals paroxysms of intense suffering.

Lyco: Violent type of gall-stone colic. Liver region rightly sensitive to touch. Constipation.

Corduus marianus : Gall-stones: Jaundice; Uncomfortable fullness in liver region; liver region sensitive to pressure. The mother tincture of the drug is to be used in 5-drops doses.

Cholesterinum: A substance which is abundantly loud in bile and billiard calculi. It is a nosade, and has been found efficacious in relieving gall-stone colic, 2X, 3X, 2 or 3 tritution. Has been used with success in this affection.

Mag-ph: (3X, 6X trit.) When administered with warm water, often relieves gall-stone colic.

Nux-v: Gall-stones and jaundice. Liver region sensitive to touch and movement. Aversion to food.

GANGRENE

Decomposition of a part of the body, there being no vitality in the part affected. In dry gangrene the parts become hard, dry, shrivelled, lack perception and assume a livid hue. Gangrene is the first stage of mortification which is destruction of all vital functions.

Therapeutics Leading Indication

Anth: Horribly offensive gangrenous ulcers. *Terrible burning, not relieved by Arsen. Though indicated.

Arsen: The parts burn like fire, look black and smell fetid. Very useful in gangrene of old persons, the gangrene being dry and better from warmth. Gangrene on tongue.

Carb-an: Ulceration, gangrene and foul-discharges. Parts bluish; indurate. Burning pains.

Crotal: Especially indicated in broken-down constitutions. Gangrene from blood-poisoning. Crotal. has the reputation of restoring vitality of parts apparently dead. Affected parts dark or bluish. Caused by mechanical injury.

Lach: In impending gangrene. Gangrenous blisters bluish or black, with burning and itching. Discharge is offensive. Gangrenous wounds, blisters, with inflammatory fever gangrene from blood-poisoning.

Secale: Dry gangrene, *esp.* in old men. Skin withered; better from cold; aggravation from external heat. *Sensation of creeping or as if ants were crawling in the affected parts. No sensation in the parts.

GASTRALGIA

Characterized by occasional pain in stomach, which is often violent and frequently associated with anaemia, tuberculosis, disorder of the liver, spleen, pancreas, stomach, ulcer or cancer of stomach etc.

Therapeutics Leading Indications

Anac: Pain in stomach only when it is empty, relieved by eating.

Arg-n: Pains worse after eating. Pains radiate from stomach to all directions, Relieved from hard pressure and bending double. Often increase and decrease gradually as in the case of Starnum.

Bell: Pressing pain, compelling the patient to bend backwards and held his breath.

Bism: Vomits as soon as the least food touches the stomach. Pains in stomach extend into the spine, relieved by bending backwards.

Bryon: Pressure of a load in stomach. Pains felt one or two hours after eating, continue for a few hours and the gradually decline. Pains worse from least motion.

Cham: Food lies in stomach like a load or stone. Pains worse at night; restlessness with anguish; better by bending double. Immediate relief from drinking a cup of coffee.

Coloc: Relief from hard pressure and bending double.

Graph: Periodical gastralgia with vomiting of food immediately after eating. Radiating pain.

Lyco: Constant fermentation of gas in abdomen, with rambling and croaking. Pains radiate from stomach to back, chest, region of ribs etc. Liver painful to touch.

Nux-v: Caused by tea, coffee, sexual excesses. Pains worse from light but relief from hard pressure. Pressure in stomach an hour or two after eating as from a stone (immediately after: Kali-bi., Nux-m.).

Phas: Burning pains relieved by external by cold and rest. Empty, hollow feeling in stomach.. Vomiting by mouthfuls without nausea, Large, hard liver.

Puls: Bad taste in mouth, *esp.* early in morning. Nourishment, whatever the kind may be, does not test nice or has no taste at all. Thirstlessness, although pain may be violent and lips may be dry. Sensation as of a stone in pit of stomach.

Ignat: Weak, empty feeling in pit of stomach not relieved by eating.

Plum: Excruciating pain in stomach. The abdomen may be retracted (drawn in or feel as if retracted), with sensation as though abdomen and backbone met. Pains in fits. Jaundice. Liver disorder.

Ver-a: Severe gastralgia an hour or two after a meal, causing thirst; radiates all over abdomen, sometimes to back and shoulder; *cold sweat on forehead. Pains may increase and decrease slowly.

GASTRITIS

Inflammation of the Stomach

Therapeutics Leading Indication

Acon: Characteristic fever. Bilious vomiting, greenish. Gagging and retching. Pressure in stomach as from a hard stone. Watery stools with pain in bowels.

Apis: Burning heat in stomach, with great soreness of the abdominal walls and vomiting (of bile).

Arnic: After mechanical injuries. Tympanitic distension of abdomen. Vomiting of coagulated blood of a deep colour. After drinking (or eating), vomiting of what has been taken, after with a mixture of blood. Eructation's as well as flatus smelling like rotten eggs. Stools are of undigested matter. *Sore bruised feeling all over.

Arsen: Heat and burning in stomach, with sharp shooting pain. Vomiting of what has been eaten or drunk. Rapid prostration of strength.

Bell: Soreness of whole abdomen, as if everything in it was excoriated and raw. Retching and violent vomiting. Pains may appear and disappear suddenly. Head hot, while the hands and feet are cold.

Bryon: The least pressure on the pit of stomach is insupportable. Eating causes extreme pain in the stomach. Which is sensitive to slight pressure Sensation of burning in stomach. Nausea and faintness of sitting up. Vomiting immediately after eating or drinking. Lips parched and dry; infrequent but copious drinking of water. *Wants to remain perfectly quiet.

Canth: Pain is stomach on being touched, as if it were ulcerated. Severe burning in stomach. *Constant desire to urinate with scanty emissions. Stools like scrapings from intestines.

Ipec: Where nausea and vomiting are remarkably pronounced. Diarrhoeal with grass-green stools and cutting colic.

Phos: Pains in stomach relieved by cold food or drink (*esp.* ice-water). Cannot tolerate least pressure on stomach even of bed-clothes. Burning in stomach, extending to throat and intestines. *Empty hollow feeling in stomach (entire abdomen) feels weak and empty). Cutting pains in stomach in fits.

Ver-a: Extreme anguish in pit or stomach. Violent nausea and vomiting. Coldness of whole body. *Cold sweat on forehead. Profound prostration. Frequent, greenish, water, gushing, exhausting stool. Intense thirst for cold drinks.

GASTRIC ULCER, DUODENAL ULCER

Gastric ulcer is more common in women than in men, whereas duodenal ulceration is more commonly met with in men than in women. The most distinctive symptom in the case of duodenal ulceration is that the pain is worse when the stomach is empty, and is relieved by taking food. For this peculiar symptom we have two remedies that stand out as supreme in both proving and results. Compare the indications of the remedies mentioned tender Gastritis, Gastralgia and Haematemesis.

Therapeutics Leading Indication

Arg-n: Small spot between xyphoid and naval sensitive to pressure; pains radiate in all directions. Gnawing, ulcerative pain in epigastrium. "Pain below and to the left of the xyphoid process in a small spot extending to a corresponding point in spine, where pressure aggravates it. Looks as if dying (Raue).

Aresen: Vomiting of blackish and brownish substances due to decomposed (blood) intense burning pains in stomach. Always worse after eating or drinking. Anaemic, of pale face.

Hydras: Vomits all the eats except milk and water mixed. Backache (may be severe). Tired aching across small of back. Excessive sweat of armpits and genitals which is offensive. *Sinking, gone feeling in stomach. Obstinate constipation.

Ignuat: Pain is located in a small circumscribed spot. Relief from eating. Pains may appear gradually and subside suddenly; or appear as suddenly as they disappear (Pains may shoot upward). Weak, empty feeling in stomach, not relieved by eating.

Kali-bi: Deep ulcers. Burning in stomach and pain of stomach; vomiting may be either sour of bitter, mix with clear mucus; of pinkish glairy fluid. "Vomits caused by every attempt to eat or drink, with distorted and burning rawness about stomach." Pressure and heaviness in stomach immediately after eating.

Kreos: Hardness in epigastrium region, with painful sensibility to touch. Stomach weak, cannot digest, food is immediately ejected or vomited some hours after eating. Burning pains in stomach. Putrid secretions. Malignancy.

Lyco: Yellowish-gray colour of face. Pit of stomach swollen and sensitive to touch. Aching in stomach in evening and after eating. No pain at night when in bed.

Phos: Gushing out of food by mouthfuls without nausea Vomiting of blood, mixed with bile and mucus. Vomiting of black substances like coffee grinds. Cold drink vomited as soon as they become warm in stomach.

Nit-ac: Stomach feels tense after a moderate meal undigested and offensive stool. Putrid smell from mouth. Pricking pains in stomach.

GLANDS, AFFECTIONS OF

Therapeutics Leading Indications

Amm-c: Painful swelling of glands of neck and of armpits. Neck glands are felt as lumps. Malignancy.

Anth: Glands painfully swollen. Glands under armpits of sub-maxillary (under jaw) glands.

Aur-met: Affects various glands. Painful swelling of the sub maxillary glands. Swelling and suppuration of inguinal glands from syphilis. Swollen neck glands.

Badi: Scrofulous swelling of glands of left side of face, throat and neck; some hard, some suppurating.

Bar-c: Infants with tonsillitis and inflamed neck glands. Glands around ears painful and swollen. Bar-c, not only swells and indurate glands, but also wastes them away. Wasting of mammary glands. Wasting of testicles.

Brom: Scrofulous or tuberculosis enlargement and in duration of glands, *esp*. on lower jaw.

Colc-f: Stony hard glands.

Clem: Swelling of sub-maxillary glands with hard nodosities (tubercles).

Coni: Glandular enlargement and in duration of stony hardness; usually painless. "Lumps and nodules indurate and enlarged glands from under the skin all over the body." Progressive debility.

Hepar: Glands of neck, groin, exilla etc. swell, become hardened and have the tendency to suppurate. Extreme sensitiveness to touch. Pricking pains.

Phyl: Glands in armpits enlarged. Sub-maxillary and parotid glands inflamed. Pains have the tendency radiate over surrounding parts.

Rhus-t: Swelling of glands (inguinal, parotid) with pain, relieved by continued motion (my experience.) I met with a case like this; Painful swelling of parotid glands (rigid side) with fairly rigid neck, pain and stiffness being relieved by continued movement of the neck to and fro, and threatened suppuration yielded to a single dose of Rhust-t., as if by the touch of a magic wand. It is for my readers to utilize this modality of Rhus-t. In any glandular affection and verify its reliability.

Silic: Indurations and swelling of scrofulous glands with or without indurations. The glands that are particular affected are cervical, parotid, axillary and inguinal one sometimes attended by troublesome itching.

Spong: Almost all the glands may be affected. The gradually enlarge and as they do, gradual increase of hardness is noticed. In all glandular swellings that the heart is affected, sponge is often the remedy. In few cases, I selected the remedy simply because the patient have suffocating spells at night. Sponge. at once cured all such cases.

Syph: Enlargement of glands in various parts of the body, particularly abundant about neck; indurent and slightly painful, causing a sensation of fullness and suffusion in face, throat and head.

Thuja: Enlargement of cervical glands. Stitching tearing pains in glands. Stitching in region of head.

Tuberculinurn: Tubercular glands of neck.

GLAUCOMA

An insidious disease characterized by increased tension within the eyeball and gradual dimness of vision.

Therapeutics Leading Indications

Bell: Excessive intolerance of light; redness of eyes and itching; throbbing.

Bryon: Eyes feel as if pressed out, often with sharp smoothing pains through eyes and head. Eyes feel sore to touch and on moving them. Increased tension of eyeball.

Coloc: Severe burning aching pain always relieved by pressure; worse from rest at night and from stooping when it feels as if it would fall out.

Kali-i: Incipient glaucoma in syphilitic subjects; vision dim and foggy; burning in eyes.

Phos: Halo round light; various lights, colours (*esp.* red), flashing before eyes. Tight pulling sensation. Black tots before eyes and diminished vision, better in twilight. Decided and unbearable nocturnal aggravation.

Physostigma: With tension in eyes which is relieves, sharp shooting pains. As if something were creeping in eyes.

Prunnus spinosa: Shooting pain from within out, or from before back wards.

Spig: Great soreness of eyes, can scarcely bear a touch. Severe pains; feels as if eye would be pressed out of the socket.

GLEET

The fourth and the last stage of gonorrhoea which is chronic in character, and which is generally attended with no pain and is characterized by the persistence of the obstinate, the transparent discharge, or sometimes this is whitish, or thick and yellowish discharge from the urethra. If often bids defiance to all treatment. It is, however, amenable to homoeopathic treatment.

Therapeutics Leading Indications

Agnus: Gleet without sexual desire or erections, yellow discharge; penis so relaxed the voluptuous find excite no erection; sexual desire lessened, almost in persons who frequently had gonorrhoea.

Nit-ac: In bad cases; after abuse of mercury, urine has intolerable, offensive, strong smell. *Pricking pain in urethra.

Sepia: Scanty discharge in morning only; meatus is glad together in morning. Discharge is yellowish; painless. Night a drop or two may stain linen yellow. Flaccid of the organs and frequent seminal emissions. If sepia fails, Kali-i. will dry up the discharge.

Silic: Sepia and Silic. have cured long-lasting gleet. Silic. has slight, shreddy discharge.

Sulph: Old cases which have not yielded to apparent indicated remedies. In sulphur constitution.

Thuja: Cutting pain at close of urination. Forked stream urine. As if a drop of urine is trickling down urethra. Last symptom is highly characteristic.

GOITRE

Chronic enlargement of the thyroid gland.

Therapeutics Leading Indication

Brom: Enlargement and indurations of thyroid gland. Goitre of the size of hen's egg.

Calc-c: Swelling is hard; worst towards new moon, scrofulous persons.

Calc-f: Gland indurate; of stony hardness.

Phyt: Modulated goitre.

Spong: Thyroid gland is swollen and hard, with suffocative attacks at night. Stitching pains and pressure. Goitre causes asthma. Pain on swallowing.

Thyroidinum: Goitre, *esp.* in fat persons, and when the swelling is brawny. Anaemia and debility. Thyr. 3X may be used, 2 or 3 doses per day and then repeated after some intervals. *Esp.* medicated in those who are anaemic, profoundly depressed, suffer from muscular weakness and palpitations from least exertion, and whose legs are oedematous. The patient is always chilly. The effect can easily be recognized by the increase of body heat.

GUMS, AFFECTIONS OF

Therapeutics Leading Indications

Ant-c: Gums stand off from teeth and bleed easily. Toothache from decayed teeth.

Arg-n: Gums tender and bleed easily but neither painful nor swollen. Gums swollen, inflamed, bleed easily and painful when touched.

Arsen: Swollen bleeding gums, painful to touch, Burning in gums. Jerking toothache at night, extending to temple.

Bar-c: Gums swollen, pale red, bleed, painful to touch. Gums swollen around a hollow tooth.

Bell: Painful swelling of gums with heat and pulsations.

Borax: Gum-boil paining severely; swelling of cheek and whole left side of face.

Carb-v: Gums spongy, bleed easily, as when touching stitching them. Gums loosened from teeth and retracted. Gums painfully sensitive when chewing.

Hepar: Swelling and inflammation of gums, which is very painful to touch. Gums ulcerate.

Kreos: Gums bluish red, soft, spongy, bieed readily. Very painful. Scorbittic, ulcerated.

Lach: Gums swollen, spongy, easily bleeding, painful. Bluish or dark purple.

Ham-ma: Profuse venous blood comes out without much of any effort, like a warm current from chest. Associated with tickling cough (expelled after a hacking cough, arnica.).

Ipec: Copious bleeding from lungs, preceded by bubbling in chest and accompanied by nausea. Blood frothy; bright red blood coming out by least effort, without cough.

Millef: Profuse flow of bright red blood, without fever; bubbling sensation in chest as if warm blood is ascending (Ipec.). In tuberculosis or incipient phthisis; patient feels unconcerned about his state and no pain with the bleeding. After injury.

Phos: When associated with dry, light, fatiguing cough, bleeding profuse and frequent, pouring out freely and then ceasing for a time. Vicarious haemoptysis for the menses. Tubercular diathesis.

Puls: Following scanty or suppression of menses; Blood black and coagulated; weakness and pain in lower part of chest; chilliness even in a warm room.

Cact: With strong throbbing of heart and sensation of constriction as of an iron-band around chest; no anxiety and no fever.

Elaps: Blood dark in colour, almost black; taste of blood in mouth.

HAEMATURIA (HAEMORRHAGE URINARY ORGANS)

Therapeutics Leading Indications

Apis: Burning soreness when urinating; stinging in urethra, urine bloody.

Arnic: Emission of blood from urethra; due to mechanical injury.

Cact: Haematuria; urination prevented by clots.

Canth: Flow of bloody mucus from bladder. Emission of blood drop by drop.

Hamam: Haematuria caused by injuries sustained. Dull pain in renal region. Great exhaustion (out of proportion to the loss of blood); tired, aching feeling in back and lower limbs.

Merc-c: Tenesmus of bladder; urine bloody; brown, with brick-dust sediment. Along with dysentery.

Puls: With burning in orifice of urethra and constrictions in region of navel. Haematuria in cows.

Tereb: Strangury, blood thoroughly mixed with urine; sediment like coffee-grounds. Much blood with very little urine. Difficult urination with burring in bladder.

HEAD, CONGESTION OF BLOOD TO

Therapeutics Leading Indications

Acon: In recent cases. On rising from recumbent position, the red face becomes pale, feels giddy.

Arg-n: Fullness of blood vessels and throbbing all over the body.

Bell: Hot and red face, sparkling eyes. Headache with violent throbbing, increased by stooping, lying down, noise or light.

Calc-c: In chronic cases; often called for after Bell. with icy coldness of hands and feet.

Gels: Congestion less violent than that of Bell. Great drowsiness. *Great heaviness of head, relieved by profuse urination. Headache begins in occiput and extends over head.

Glon: *Esp.* when caused by exposure to rays of sun. From suppressed menses (Puls.). Sudden rush of blood to head and violent congestion; bursting, throbbing headache; violent action of heart.

Hyos: Often required after Bell. with delirium, unconsciousness, yet the patient answers all questions properly. Face red, purple.

Kali-c: Violent ebullition of blood with throbbing in all arteries. May be associated with oppressed breathing.

Nux-v: When caused by mental overwork or use of liquors, coffee or opium, sexual excesses.

Opium: *Bluish red and bloated face. *Stupor, snoring, rattling. Cold sweat on face.

Puls: Sensation of heat on head, relieved by cold application.

Phos: Heat on top of head, Congestion spreads from spine to head. Congestions often painful. Washing clothes or walking fast causes rush of blood to the head. Chronic congestion of head.

Sulph: *Constant heat on top of head; Cold feet; frequent flashings. After suppression of cutaneous eruptions.

HEADACHE

Therapeutics Leading Indications

Acon: Sensation as if whole brain would start out of eyes. Violent stupefying headache with sensation of fullness.

Arsen: Periodical headache. Headache relieved by cold application for a moment, returning much more strongly afterwards. With vomiting after eating, drinking. Anxious. Restless.

Act-r: With great pain in eyebolls. Feels as if going crazy with headache. Rush of blood to head, brain feeling too large for the cranium. As if brain is moving in waves. Headache of students.

Bell: With red face, throbbing pain, *esp.* in forehead, obliging one to close eyes. Cannot bear noise or bright light. Headache *worse from lying down. Better from pressure, tight bandaging, wrapping up. Head hot, feel cold.

Bryon: Worse from *slightest motion; *wants to lie perfectly still. When stooping, brain feels as if it would burst through her forehead. Commences in morning, gradually increasing until evening. Begins in morning after opening eyes (not simply on waking), and may last till evening. Pain in head always shifts to the side lain on. Pain relieved by pressure. Caused by constipation. Thirst for large quantities of water.

Cact: Begins in morning and grows worse as day advances. Violent neuralgia in right side of head; periodic.

Cham: Goes almost furious with pain. *One cheek red, the other pale, bitter bilious vomiting.

China: From suppressed crazy. Intense throbbing headache after haemorrhage or sexual excess. Neuralgic headache, periodical, on alternate days (Ambra.) often changing sides. As skull would burst. Worse on sitting or lying, must stand or walk.

Coccul: Intense headache in occipital region, in lower point of back of head, and in nape of neck. Pains in back of head as if is were alternately opening and closing. Occipital headache with inability to lie on back of head.

Coff: Headache intolerable, driving to despair or making one tearful. As if a nail were driven in brain. Extreme wakefulness.

Gels: Headache with soreness of eyes on moving there (Bryon.). Cannot fix his attention to anything. Gets blind before headache comes on. Head feels enlarged. A great remedy for occipital headache.

Glon: Sunstroke and headache from recent exposure to the sun. Headache increases and decreases everyday with the sun. Throbbing and feeling of fullness. Great sensitive ness to least jar. Head feels as if enlarged, distended. Headache in place of menses.

Ignat: Pain as if nail were driven out through side of head, Pain changes locality. Pain comes on gradually and abate suddenly (Sulph-ac.); or comes and goes suddenly (Bell.). Better from warmth and lying on painful side. Relief from profuse flow on colourless urine.

Ipec: With Nausea and vomiting. Pain in head (skull) extends downwards to teeth.

Iris-v: Hemi crania (headache confined to one side of head) *begins with blurring of sight. Of gastric origin or from liver troubles. Sour, watery vomiting. Worse from rest, better from moderate motion. Right-sided headache, beginning with a blur and very severe in front of head.

Kali-bi: *Blurred vision or blindness precedes headache (Gels. & Lac-d.). Pain settles in one small spot, which can be covered with the point of a finger. Pains appear and disappear suddenly, shift from one place to another.

Kalm: Very useful in sun headache (headache comes on at sunrise, gradually gets worse till noon, when it is at its height, declines as sun gets down). Right-sided headache. Begins in occipital and runs up; affects also face worse right side.

Lach: Headache from heat of sun. Headache every morning on awaking. One-sided (*esp.* Left-sided) headache; worse in and over left eye. Headache *begins in left side and extends to right. * Worse after sleep. Cannot bear to have hair touched.

Mag-p: Neuralgic headache; pains sharp, cutting, shooting or stitching; intermittent; unbearable; changing places; relieved by warmth and pressure.

Nat-m: School girls' anaemic headache (Calc-p.). Headaches which appear periodically with great severity; head feels as it bursting. Chronic, periodical, Semi-lateral, from sunrise to sunset, with pale face, nausea, vomiting. Headache begins with partial blindness (Iris, Kali-bi). Pains intermitting. Headache causing by dye-stain (Ruta) malarial headache always worse at sea-side.

Nux-v: Headache every morning on waking; after eating worse during motion, even when turning eyes. From mental exertion; masturbation.

Petrol: A valuable remedy for obstinate occipital headache occiput feels as heavy as lead. Throbbing occipital headache head feeling numb, as if it were made of wood and bruised this throbbing is a keynote.

Phos: Neuralgic headache; head must be kept warmly wrapped up day and night. Accumulation of much saliva during headache. Washer woman's headache.

Phos-ac: Headache of school children (Nat-m.); constant dull depressing pain with blurring of vision; pains disappear during vacation, reappearing when studies and resumed. Headache of school-girls from eye-strain and resumed and of overuse of eyes (Calc-p., Nat-m., Ruta). Crushing weight on vertex, from long—lasting grief or nerve exhaustion.

Phyt: Headache of syphilitic origin. Intense headache and backache. Worse from moving.

Pic-ac: Headache worse from artificial light, least overcall excitement. Sensation as in rain were too large for cranium.

Puls: *Esp.* in case of women, with scanty menses and disposition to weep easily. Pains extend to ear and teeth. Pains shift from one place to another, often *rapidly. Worry in evening; from warmth. Relief in open air and by bandaging.

Rhus-t: When brain feels loose, as if striking against skull on walking, rising or shaking,... When caused be sitting or lying in cold; better from warmth and motion.

Sang: A valuable remedy in hemicranias affection right-side. *Right-sided headache, pain begins in occiput, spreding upwards and settles over right eye. Periodic; every seventh day. Increases and decreases with course of sun, evidence reaching at midday. Bursting headache, as if eyes, to be pressed out. Sleeping relieves.

Mell: Violent congestive headache with red face shot eyes, throbbing carotids and finally nosebleed relieves.

Selen: Of rakes and drunkards. Headache, weakness, great sadness, irritability etc. follow seminal in Pain over left eye; *worse weakling in sun; worse from tea. Fatigued from hot weather.

Sulph: Sick headache every week or every two week very weakening, with heat on top of head and coldness of free flushes in face.

HEARING, DEFECTS OF

Therapeutics Leading Indications

Arnic: Hardness of hearing from blows, concussions; discharge of blood from ears, from nose.

Bar-c: Hearing impaired from chronic enlargement tonsils.

Calc-c: Chronic hardness of hearing, *esp.* after suppression of intermittent fever by quinine. From working in water Deafness in childhood.

Carb-an: Hearing confused; does not know from what direction sound comes; *swelling of periosteum behind ear.

Caust: Sound re-echoes unpleasantly, even his own sound. Words and steps re-echo in his or her ears, sudden re-echoing causing difficulty in hearing.

China: Hardness of hearing, humming and roaring in ears. From loss of animal fluids.

Gels: Nervous deafness of mild form; sudden loss or hearing for a short time.

Graph: Hardness of hearing, better when riding is a carriage, *where in a noise.

Kreos: Deafness from hereditary syphilis Humming and hardness of hearing before and during menses.

Lach: "Hardness from hereditary, with want of cerumen partially relieved by inserting fingers in external meatus and shaking it.****" (Lilienthal).

Nit-ac: Hardness of hearing from indurations and swelling of tonsils. Hardness of hearing but hears better when riding in a carriage. One's own speech echoes in ears.

Puls: Hardness of hearing as if ears were stopped. Hears better when riding in a carriage.

Silic: Stoppage of ears which open at times with a loud report. Oversensitive to laud sounds.

Sulph: Deafness, *esp.* for human voice. Eating aggravates deafness.

Verbascum: Has reputation for curing many cases of deafness. Deafness as from stoppage of ears (first left, then right) while reading aloud. (Verbascum Thapsus a commonly known as Great Mullein. The well known Mullein oil is of much use in deafness and *esp.* in earache. Two or three drops of the oil may be instilled into ears night and morning for deafness. The author has, however, no experience in the matter.)

HAIR, FALLING OF

Therapeutics Leading Indications

Bar-c: Losing of hair from crow. Baldness.

Flaor-ac: Hair splits and breaks. (In my hand a case has cured by a single dose of the remedy in the 10th potency.) Kent writes;

"If examined closely under the microscope, it is seen to be necroses, little ragged ulcers will be found along the course of the hair."

Kali-c: Dryness and rapidly falling off of hair with much dandruff.

Sepia: Great falling off of hair; scalp and roots of hair very sensitive to touch; much itching of scalp.

Baldness: The three great remedies in baldness are: Bald Lyco., Silic. Bar-c. has losing of hair from crown of the Lyco. Has gained reputation from the experience of Jahr. Silic. Is indicated in premature baldness. Develops and, therefore, cures complete bladness on Sepia has bald spots on scalp Flour-ac, is useful in dandruf developed from hairs which break off.

HEART, PALPITATION OF

Therapeutics Leading Indications

Acon: When caused by fright or overexertion, anxiety and fear of death.

Arnic: After straining heart from violent running.

Arsen: Violent palpitation of heart, *esp.* at night, visible audible, with anguish; cannot lie on back.

Bell: Violent palpitation reverberating to head. On top of head, coldness of feet.

Coff: After excessive joy, surprise.

Digit: Sensation as if heart would stop beating. If one moved. Palpitation excited on going up slight ascent, by talking, and at each movement of body.

Ferr-m: Palpitation better from walking slowly. Throbbing in all blood vessels. Anaemia. Soft bellows-sound at apex of heart.

Kali-c: Palpitation in spells taking away breath, impending suffocation with inability to lie down.

Lach: Palpitation with choking from slightest anxiety. Can bear not pressure on throat and chest must sit up or lie on right side.

Lyco: *Esp.* during digestion or in bed nearly every evening, at times attended with anxiety and trembling.

Nux-v: From alcoholic liquors, coffee, highly seasoned food.

Opium: After alarming events, causing fright, grief. Drown etc.

HAEMORRHOIDS, PILES

Therapeutics Leading Indication

Aesc: Sensation of dryness and heat in rectum; as rectum is full of small sticks which prick the mucous membrane (Collin.). Piles painful, burning, itching. Purplish rarely bleeding. *Severe and constant dull backache affecting sacrum and hips.

Aloe: Protruding piles like a bunch of grapes, blue constant bearing down in rectum; bleeding, sore, tender hot, relieved by cold water, Intense itching. Much emision of flatus before stool.

Arsen: Blind (not bleeding) piles with burn like for particularly at night. All symptoms worse after midnight.

Collin: Chronic, painful, bleeding piles. Sensation as sticks, sand or gravel has lodged in rectum (Aesc.).

Hamam: Profuse bleeding with marked soreness. Piles in flamed, Bluish, Back feels as if it would break.

Ignat: Pain and bleeding are worse when stool is loose tumor protrudes from slight exertion at stool. Shots stitches from anus deep into rectum. Cutting and tears pains in rectum continuing for hours after stool.

Lach: Protruding piles with stitches, felt *esp.*, during cold or sneeze, which generally shoot upwards (Nit-ac.). Bears in anus, as with little hammers. Tumor bluish.

Nux-v: Blind or bleeding piles. Stitching, burning or itching in rectum and anus. Sensation of constriction in rectum. Frequent but ineffectual urging to stool.

Ratan: Great protrusion of piles; *Followed for a long time by burning in anus. Straining at Stool extorts crying. Stool, pain as if from splinters of glass. Embedded in anus and rectum.

Sulph: Blind, bleeding or moist piles flowing dark blood tingling, burning, and soreness in and about a Frequent ineffectual urging to stool. Constipation.

Carb.v: Bluish; oozing of very fetid imposture.

Podo: Piles and prolepses of rectum with Stool or from least motion.

Sepia: Difficulty in passing stool, which seems to stick in anus or rectum as if a ball or potato were there.

Mur-ac: Piles inflamed and swollen; bluish; violent stitches. Piles appear suddenly in children.

HERNIA

Protrusion of some of the contents of the abdomen through the abdominal walls causing a swelling is called Hernia. Protrusions at the navel, in the groin, and in the scrotum are respectively called umbilical. Inguinal and total Hernia. Hernia is reducible when it can be readily returned into the abdomen, irreducible, when it cannot be returned; strangulated, when it is not only incapable of being returned, but also when there is in addition pain, constriction and inflammation, with nausea, vomiting, febrile symptoms etc.

Therapeutics Leading Indication

Acon: When inflammation had commenced in the strangulated bowels, Soreness, burning and heat in affected part. Extreme sensitiveness to contact.

Amm-c: Hernia in left Groin.

Aur-met: Protrusion of inguinal hernia, sometimes; with cramp-like pains. Inguinal and umbilical hernia of children caused by crying.

Bell: "Soon after strangulation which is caused by spasmodic action of the muscular fibers and before inflammation has set in." (Raue)

Coccul: When protrusion takes place very slowly, as if from paralytic state of abdominal ring. Tendency to protrusion of inguinal hernia. The least jar is unbearable. Painful with inclination to hernia, *esp.* after rising from sitting.

Lach: Skin covering hernia tumor is livid. Coughing and sneezing go like knife through the tumor. Hernia exceedingly sensitive to touch; will not admit handling (Bell,. Nux-v.). When gangrene threatens strangulated hernia.

Lyco: *Esp*. indicated in hernia of right side.

Nux-v: Strangulated hernia. Sudden violent pain in hernial region. It is a valuable remedy for inguinal and umbilical hernia. When there is a feeling of weakness in abdomen, particularly in region of inguinal canal, in morning on rising. Slow protrusion (Caccul.) in aged persons. Left side mostly affected.

Plumb: It has in many cases resolved strangulation where Acon., Bell., and Nux-v. failed. Incarcerated hernia. Vomiting containing fecal matters. Violent colic.. Inflammation and gangrene of bowels.

Rhus-t: When caused by straining or lifting heavy weight. Efficacious in hernia of recent occurrence.

Sulph-ac: Very efficacious in inguinal hernia. Violent hiccough. Sensation of trembling all over body, without trembling.

Thuja: Very useful in *left-sided inguinal hernia. Sweats only on covered parts, while uncovered parts are dry and hot.

Borax: Infantile hernia. Child dreads downward motion has anxious countenance when carried downstairs. Family frightened.

Calc-c: Infantile hernia. Rachitic children; big-bellied perspire; about head when sleeping.

Opium: When face is dark red, with soporus condition; constipation.

Ver-a: In dangerous cases associated with hiccough. Cold sweat (*esp*. *on forehead), nausea with sensation of fainting and violent thirst.

HICCOUGH

Therapeutic Hints

Simple cases often yield to Nux-v.

After cold drinks: Nux-v.

From overeating or from tobacco: Nux-v.

Worse from least motion: Bryon.
With sour belching and flatulency: China.
Loud-sounding dangerous hiccough: Cicu.
With stitches in stomach: coccul.
Constant hiccough; hiccough for hours at a time: Cloche.
After abdominal operation: Hyos.
Violent hiccough at night: Hyos.
Frequent and violent hiccough with profuse flow of saliva: Lobel.
Hiccough thirty times a minute; for sixty days, life is in danger: Magi-P. cured such a case.
Violent hiccough *esp.* in evening: Niccolum.

HOARSENESS, APHONIA

Therapeutics Leading Indications

Amm-caust: Loss of voice with burning rawness in throat.

Arg-met: Total loss of voice with speakers and professional singers. Burning and rawness in throat and larynx, worse from talking or singing.

Arg-n: Chronic aphonia. Chronic laryngitis of singers, raising of voice causing cough.

Arum-t: Hoarseness; Inflammation and irritation.

Caust: Hoarseness, burning roughness (Soreness) of throat, worse mornings, caused by dry, cold sever winter weather, dryness of larynx. Cough relieved by a drink of cold water.

Gels: Aphonic from paretic stage of laryngeal muscles; can only whisper.

Phos: Hoarseness with cough and rawness in larynx and bronchi. *esp.* Behind sternum, worse in evening, when there may be aphonic. Cannot talk on account of pain in larynx; larynx sensitive to touch (Caust, must not be used before or after Phos.).

Rhus-t: From overstraining voice.

Selen: Very useful for hoarseness of singers, especially when it comes on beginning to sing. From long-talking.

Spong: with voice cracked or faint. Sensation of a plug in larynx.

HYDROCELE

An accumulation of serous fluid either in the membrane of the scrotum, in the coats of the testicles, or in the cellular texture of the spermatic cord.

Therapeutics Leading Indications

Calc-c: In scrofulous cases with general symptoms of the drug.

Digit: Left side most affected with swelling of testicles.

Rhodo: *Esp.* when it is left-sided. Has cured cases of long-standing where no cause could be found and where there was no disease of the testes. Hydrocele in child, from birth, right-sided. Smooth, hard swelling on left side. From birth, increasing from year to year.

Puls: Of congential form. Dropsically swelling of Scrotum of a whitish blue colour.

When caused by mechanical injury and contusion; Arnic., Coni. From excessive sexual indulgence: Coni. Dropsy of scrotum and prepuce; hydrocele: Apis. After gonorrhoeal rachitic, with sexual weakness: Phos. Of long-standing, large swelling of scrotum, containing dark, thick fluid, throbbing: Hepar.

In acute hydeocele: Apis, or Hellebores is apt to cause absorption of the fluid.

HYDROCEPHALUS

Accumulation of watery fluid within the cranium (brain), which may be congenital or acquired. It is characterized by enlargement of the skull, wider fontanelles and bones of skull feeling thin under pressure of the fingers.

Therapeutics Leading Indication

Apis: Boring head into pillow. Profuse sweat on head, of musk-like odour. Scanty urine. *Sudden, shrill, piercing cry while the child is asleep.

Apoc: Head large; bulging of frontal bones. Sutures wide open. Stupor with constant involuntary motion of one arm and leg. One eye motionless, the other rolling.

Bar-c: Psoric or tubercular diathesis. Child idiotic. Memory deficient. Swelling and indurations of glands, *esp.* cervical and inguinal.

Calc-c: Fat babies having large head with wide open fontanel's; profuse sweat on head while sleeping, *esp.* on occiput.

Calc-p: Children emaciated; scrofulous: unable to stand; sunken, flabby abdomen; skull thin and brittle; posterior fontanel's wide open; neck weak, unable to support head; delayed dentition congenital form.

Hell: After exudation has taken place. Child lies wholly unconscious. Muscles of forehead corrugated. Constant chewing motion of jaw. Automatic motion of one arm and one leg. When offered, drinks greedily from nervousness. Bores head into pillows; rolls head. Urine dark and scanty, loaded with albumen.

Hyos: Stupor or complete loss of consciousness. When spoken to answer properly, but immediately stupor returns. *Picking at bed-clothes (Bell., Strum.). Cries out suddenly (Apis., Bell.).

Lyco: Child apparently sleepy, but screams out suddenly in sleep, stares about and cannot easily be pacified.

Silic: Rickety children; profuse sweat about head at night, *esp.* forehead and face. Fetid sweet of feet.

Thuj: Children of sycotic or syphilitic taint. Their parents (one or both), have a greasy skin *esp.* of face, warts, decaying roots or sordes of teeth, crowns remaining sound, sweat only in covered parts have dropsically bloated face. The child is apt to develop these hereditary symptoms.

Calc-c: From masturbation or other sexual excesses (Nux-v., Sulph.). Sexual powers (erections) diminished emission too quick or imperfect. Great prostration after coition followed by trembling and weakness. Sexual gratification is followed by vertigo, headache and weakness in knees; also confusion of ideas in worst cases.

Conium: From *suppressed sexual appetite or from over-indulgence. Sexual desire without erections. "Emission on the slightest stimulus, such as merely being in the society of women." Emission without creations. *Esp.* in old and old bachelors. Useful in strong, healthy men who have great desire but no erection and who have an emission as soon as they begin to caress a woman."

Lyco: Reputed to be one of the best remedies for importance. Erections imperfect or absent. In "old men who marry again but find themselves impotant.' Young men who become impotent from masturbation or sexual excess. Old men with strong desire but imperfect erections.

Nux-v: Bad effects of masturbation; of sexual excesses, Spermatorrhoea. Nervous, irritable persons with gastric disturbance.

Selen: Coldness and relaxation or sexual organs. Oozing of prostatic fluid during sleep, at stool, and after urination. Erections slow, insufficient, two rapid emission, with long continued thrill; weakness, mental confusion, headache, irritability following sexual emission. Semen thin and odourless.

Staph: From self-abuse or sexual excesses. Sunken features; guilty, abashed facial expression, loss of memory; sadness; nocturnal emissions; backache; weak legs, lustreless eyes; sexual organs relaxed. In worst case atrophy of the organs.

Thuja: *Impotence after gonorrhoea.

Anac: Loss of confidence; afraid to marry for fear of impotency.

Gels: Organs relaxed, cold, and sexual power exhausted, lightest excitement causing emissions.

INFLUENZA

Therapeutics Leading Indications

Acon: High fever with dry skin; restlessness; great thirst.

Arsen: Profuse fluent coryza with discharge of burning, excoriating water; great debility; constipation. Great thirst, drinks often but little at a time, violent sneezing.

Bapt: A very valuable remedy in epidemic influenza according to my experience in hundreds of cases. Great languor: soreness of body; feels bruised in all parts of body; wants to lie down. Chilly on going into open air.

Eup-perf: Great soreness and aching of whole body as if in bones. Pains cause restlessness without any relief from motion; cough with great soreness of trachea and chest; cough hurts head and chest; Patient holds chest with hands while coughing.

Rhus-t: Severe aching of all bones; copious coryza with redness and oedema of throat; coughing and sneezing; great restlessness; after exposure to dampness.

Sabad: Violent spasmodic sneezing shaking the whole body and Lachrymation on going into open air; Copious watery coryza; Throat swollen, pain worse on empty swallowing. Wants everything warm; sits by fire.

Bell: Hot skin, with sweat on covered parts; flushed face; severe headache, *esp.*, throbbing headache; dryness in mouth and throat; spasmodic cough; sleepy but cannot sleep.

Camph: Chilliness at the onset; body is cold both subjectively and objectively; nose dry and stopped up; death-like paleness of face.

Carb-ac: Regarded as a specific for influenza during attack in the 3X potency. Resulting debility (30th potency) in my experience, I found Baptisia 30 almost a specific for weakness following influenza. Any way Carb-ac. has cold hands and feet; profound prostration and fatigue.

Merc-s: Rheumatic pains with sore-throat, not relived by sweat; Flabby tongue taking imprint of teeth; fluent coryza with much sneezing.

Nux-v: Great heat, whole body burning hot; *esp.* face red and hot; the patient cannot move a bit or uncover in the least without feeling chilly.

Phos: Epidemic influenza; bronchial affection with dry tickling cough and tightness across chest; hoarseness, husky, rough voice; great weakness.

Sang: Crazy acrid, watery; nose sore and raw, Dry distressing cough with burning and rawness in chest. Breath and sputa smell offensive, even to the patient. Violent headache affecting the right eye.

INJURIES

Therapeutics Leading Indications

Arnic: Either acute or chronic effects of mechanics injuries. Bruises, contusions; *esp.* bruises with well-marked echymosis and concussions of brains and spine. Injuries with blunt instruments. Hemorrhages of mechanic origin whether in the tissues of internal organs or the skin strain from lifting heavy things or after over-exertion Nosebleed from mechanical injuries. Feels tired after seeing moving pictures. (I have always used the 30th and 200th potencies with desired effect.)

Calend. Invaluable as local application to clean surgical cuts or lacerated wounds in preventing excessive suppuration (Of course, it may at the same time be administered potencies to advantage.). For external wounds with or without loss of substances, *esp.* when associated will great soreness and pain. Use it both internally 30 (potencies) and externally (in watery solution, 1 dram of mother tincture diluted with 4 to 6 ounces of water. A useful haemostatic in tooth-extraction. Strains in injuries of single muscles (Ruta, Rhuts-T.). It is our great antiseptic.

Coni: Injuries to glands; indurations resulting from contusions and bruises (Sulph-ac. Follows well). Glandular indurations of stony hardness after bruises. Mechanical injuries to periosteum.

Hamam: Incised, lacerated, contused wounds, wounds from fall, and bleeding after injuries. Here it relievers soreness of muscles, relieves pain, even heals wounds and checks hemorrhage, sometimes excelling Arnica or any other remedy. Even useful in chorionic effects or mechanical injuries (Arnic., Coni.).

Hyper: *Esp.* for wound of *parts rich in sentient nerves (fingers, *Esp.* finger-ends, toes, matrices of nails, coccyx, Palms and soles). Mechanical injuries (concussion) to brain and spine. A wonderful remedy for *Punctured wounds *esp.* from stepping on nails, needles and the like (Ledum), Lacerated wounds; soreness and excruciating pain, Preserves integrity or torn and lacerated membranes when almost entirely separated from body (Calends.). Traumatic neuritis and neuralgias.

Ruta: Mechanical injuries to bones and periosteum more particularly for bruised bones with great soreness. Wounds where bones have been injured. Useful for parts indicated if tendinous parts are overstrained.

INSOMNIA, SLEEPLESSNESS

Therapeutics Leading Indication

Bell: In children *esp.* plethoric. Drawsy but cannot sleep. "On closing the eyes in order to go the sleep, frightful vision and jerking of limbs."

Calc-c: Lies awake night after night. Long wakefulness which is the precursor to some disease and the accompaniments of others." She has visions on closing eyes; starts at every little noise. During dentition.

China: After loss of blood, or any *Vital fluid and debilitating diseases. With crowding of ideas. Weakness night-sweat.

Cina: Tossing about in sleep, crying and lamentation; child will not sleep unless rocked or kept in constant motion. Wakes up trembling and frightened.

Coccul: From pure mental activities and disturbances. Great flow of ideas interrupting sleep. Wakes frequently slightest loss of sleep tells on him.

Coff: Due to excessive mental and physical excitement. The mind is active with plans, fancies and ideas. All senses more acute. (Give a dose of Coff. 200 before going to bed.).

Gels: Dull and drowsy, but cannot fall asleep. From exhaustion of nervous system.

Ignat: From grief. Suppressed mental suffering. Sensation of goneness or sinking in stomach at night, causing sleep lessness.

Nux-v: Caused by abuse of alcoholic liquors, coffee, tobacco etc. Cannot keep from falling asleep in evening hours before bedtime; lies awake for an hour or two, at 3 or 4 a.m.; then sleeps late in the morning. Awakes tired and weak with many complaints in morning, e.g., headache.

Opium: Seems sleepy but cannot sleep. Sleeplessness with acuteness of hearing. Sleep disturbed by sounds at a distance ordinarily not heard at all. Old persons; children drunkards.

Puls: Wide awake in evening. Sleep restless wide frequent waking and full of troubled and frightful dreams. From indigestion; after quinine.

Sulph: Sleepy in daytime but sleepless at night. Sleep in cat naps; slightest noise awakens him. And then great difficulty in falling asleep. Becomes suddenly wide awake at night. (In sleeplessness, Sulph. May be given at night; when given at night to one who sleeps well, sulph. May produce insomnia, which it is intended to combat.).

INTERMITTENT FEVER

In most cases due to malaria. Some are due to psoric or tubercular maism. In malaria, medicines, as a rule, require frequent repetitions. Symptoms in the cold, heat and sweat stage, in particular, determine selection.

Therapeutics Leading Indications

Apis: *Chill with thirst always; Chill worse in a warm room or from external heat. Chill about 3 p.m. renewed chilliness from slightest motion. *Oppression of chest, as if patient would smother. Heat rarely with thirst. Sweat alternating with dryness of skin. Sweat stage is usually wanting (it may be of low grade). Nat-m. is often called for after Apis has failed to complete a cure.

Arsen: Sleepy before attack chill never clearly defined; frequently intermingled with heat; better from external heat. Heat: dry burning, intense, great restlessness; insatiable thirst, drinks often but little at a time. Sweat: often wanting; if any, cold clammy. Dropsy. one *esp.*, the cold stage is wanting.

Bryon: Chill: with great thirst: violent, dry, racking cough with stitching pains in chest and region of spleen. Heat with increased thirst; wants to be quiet.

Caps: "Valuable remedy in intermittent occurring in midsummer." Before Chill there is thirst ("knows like chill in coming, because he wants to drink") but no pain Chill. With great thirst yet worse after drinking; shivering and chilliness after every drink, chill commences in back and then extends over the whole body. After chill sweat without previous heat; or after chill heat without thirst.

Charb-v: After abuse of quinine. Paroxysm irregular, sometimes commencing with sweat followed by chilliness Chill: with thirst; coldness of legs up to knees, even in bed Heat; without thirst; desire to be fanned. Sweat: profuse, sour, offensive.

China: Thirst of China is guiding. Thirst before chill (the patient surmises an attack from this thirst which is the precursor to a chill); thirst ceases as soon as chill begins (peculiarity of his thirst is that it increases from every drink); *heat without thirst, or thirst may begin at chill is over, but it decreases as heat increases, there being entire absence of thirst during height of paroxysm; when fever subsides thirst begins; *great thirst during sweat. *Fever coming on every other day.

Gels: Aching all over body; drowsy; feels tired with desire to lie down and sleep. Chill runs up and down the back; severe nervous chill though skin is warm, wants to be held so that he may not shake so much. Sweat relieves pain.

Ignat: Thirst only during chill (Ferr-m.). During heat neetle-rash over whole body.

Ipec: If no other remedy is indicated, give in heat stage a few doses of Ipec. 30 in rapid succession, say, every one hour or so, and you will find that malarial fever has been aborted. If the cure is not complete, such administration of the drug will serve to clear up the case and pave the way for some other remedy to complete the cure. If in a chronic case, relapses from dietetic irregularities take place, this remedy often comes not play. *Nausea and vomiting predominate in all stages *esp*. at one set. sweat on cepper upper parts of body. After abuse of or suppression form quinine.

Lyco: Fever worse from 4 to 8 p.m. or *paroxysm come on at about 4 p.m. and terminate at about 8 a.m. Chill; one foot hot, the other cold. Heat; with thirst for warm drinks, nausea after cold drinks; sour vomiting. Sweat immediately after chill, without intervening heat (Caust.).

Nux-v: Chill: violent, without thirst; blueness of finger nails; fingers and hands cold and bluish. *Great heat, whole body burning hot, *esp*. face red and hot, yet the patient comes move or uncover in the least without feeling chilly. A pyrexia. Bilious symptoms: paralytic weakness in legs.

Puls: Symptoms ever changing, no two paroxysms are alike. Increasing severity of attacks. Chill at 4 p.m. without thirst. Intolerable burning heat in bed, wants to be uncovered. Moans and groans; licks the lips but does not drink. One-sided sweat, sweat on the left side being characteristic. A pyrexia: Constant chilliness; Bitter taste in mouth. Thirst of Pulls, is guiding. Thirst only during heat, but it decreases as heat increases, there being entire absence of thirst during height of paroxysm, thirst beginning after the fever is over. Then again, sweat with great thirst.

Rhus-t: *Dry teasing fatiguing cough coming an hours before chill and continuing during chill. Severe chill (at 7 p.m.) as if dashed with ice-water. Heat excessive, as if hot water were running through blood-vessels. Restless, constantly changes position. Urticaria over whole body passing off during sweat stage. Pyrexia: Hydroa on upper lip.

Sepia: "Cases that have been spoiled by quinine or by bungling administration of homoeopathic remedies." "Clears up malaria diathesis in chronic cases." Intermittent fever followed by violent heat and inability to collect one's senses; this followed by profuse perspiration.

Ant-c: Gastric symptoms predominate; great sadness and woeful mood; *thick milky white coating on tongue; longing for acids, *esp*. pickles; great desire for sleep; chill predominates frequent relapse from gastric derangement.

Caust: Sweat immediately after chill, without intervening heat (Anl-t.); chilliness of whole left side of body; flushes of heat followed by chill; morning sweat (smelling sour).

Cham: *Esp*. Intermittent of children. *One cheek red and hot, the other pale and cold.

Cina: Frequently called for in epidemic intermittent in children. Canine hunger; picking nose during fever; desire for sweet things; irritable.

Iodi: Fever of intermittent type in tuberculosis patients. Indicated by general characteristic of the remedy such as; Ravenous hunger; eats freely and well, yet/loses flesh all the time.

JAUNDICE

Not a disease in itself, but a symptom of some disorder, characterized by a yellow discoloration of the skin, eyes etc., caused by absorption of bile into the blood. Consult the indications given under Liver affections and Gall stones when required.

Therapeutics Leading Indications

Acon. For acute pain in liver, clay coloured stool. Yellow yellowish colour of skin. An useful remedy for in newborn children; also during pregnancy.

Arsen: After long fever; after abuse of quinine (Nux-v.). In different liver affections. Yellowness of sclerotica (Chem., China).

Bryon: With obstinate constipation, stool dry and hard. *Lips parched, dry and cracked, Pains *esp.* stitching in liver, on being touched or coughing.

Card-m: With dull headache; white coated tongue, *esp.* in middle; nausea with vomiting of acid. Green fluid. Jaundice complicated with gallstones; uncomfortable fullness in liver region.

Cham: In newborn children. Yellowness of face and whites of eyes. Stools white, slimy, green, watery; with colic. Irritable, impatient mood. Child cries; quiet only when carried.

China: Brought on by loss of animal fluids, by sexual excesses. Skin and sclerotic (whites of eye) yellowish. Liver swollen, hard and sensitive to touch. Abdomen feels full and tight as if stuffed. Jaundice from gall-stones.

Merc-s: An important remedy, often required after Acon. Complete jaundice. Skin very yellow or dirty yellow. Sweat stains linen yellow. Clay-coloured and offensive stool. Jaundice after abuse of quinine.

Nux-v: After abuse of quinine; from too high living. In complication with gall-stone. Nausea and bilious vomiting. Frequent but ineffectual urging to stool.

Podo: Jaundice associated with gall-stone; in complication with liver affections. Dirty watery stool; offensive. Stool may be chalk-like, undigested. Liver feels as it dragged down.

Crotal: Malignant, black jaundice. Dark blood flows from nose, mouth, bowels, uterus etc.

Iodi: Dirty yellowish skin yellow, almost dark brown colour of face. Canine hunger all the time.

Phos: In complication with lung disease of deep-seated brain disease. Jaundice associated with anaemia. During pregnancy. Nervous exhaustion with general heaviness and dread of motion. Stool grayish with constant chilliness even in a warm room.

KIDNEY, AFFECTIONS OF

Two glandular bodies situated on each side of the loins having the function of secreting or separating urine from the blood. The study of the following remedies will enable the readers to treat Albuminuria (Bright's disease). And Nephritis (inflammation of the kidneys associated with morbid secretions from these organs).

Therapeutics Leading Indications

Acon: Acute nephritis. Dark, scanty urine; for retention of urine with stitches in kidneys. Characteristic fever.

Apis: Acute nephritis, albuminuria. During or after any eruptive disease. Urine scanty and loaded with albumen. Dropsy with pale, waxen skin, thirstlessness; predominates in upper part of body.

Arg-n: touching the region of the kidney excites pain; pain extends from kidneys to bladder; urine dark red. Urine contains much uric acid or deposits of uric acid crystals. Dried-up look. Urine burning while passing and urethra feels as if swollen. It resembles Cantharis and is often useful after its failure.

Arsen: General anasarea, skin pale, waxy earth-coloured. Excessive exhaustion from least exertion. Oppression of breath at night, *esp.* *after midnight and on lying down, with great anguish. Urine is scanty and aluminous. Urine looking like dark dung-water and renal casts are, abundant.

Bell: Spasmodic, crampy pains, straining along. Urethra to bladder. Pains appear and disappear suddenly. Retention of urine deposits a cloud of phosphates. Urine first clearer deep-red with white sediment. Sensation of a worm in bladder (of a ball, Lach.).

Berb: Acute pains (of various kinds) in region of kidneys. Pain extends from kidney to bladder and urethra. Pains seem to radiate in all directions from kidneys, particularly downward and forward, extending into pelvis; pains in loins and hips. Great urging to urinate with pain in neck to bladder with scanty urine. Urine may be aluminous of slimy when passed, depositing foamy yellowish sediment of depositing transparent, reddish or jelly-like sediment.

Canth: As a rule, indicated in an acute case. Nephritis associated with irritation of bladder of all grades. Violent, burning, cutting pains in neck of bladder. Urine scolds him; passed drop by drop. Constant urging to urinate; urine hot, scalding; intolerable tenesemus. Urine bloody or deep red without blood; aluminous.

Digit: Nephritis with dropsy; pulse very slow and weak; scanty urine which is dark, turbid and aluminous. Urine may be suppressed. Sudden sensation as if heart stood still.

Nax-v: Nephralgia *esp*. In right kidney, extending to genitals and right leg; pain in renal region as if a foreign body were there; pain better from lying on back; spermatic cords contracted, testicles drawn up. Painful ineffectual urging to urinate.

Ocimum ean: Has cured many cases of pain. Pain in upper part of the region of right kidney, extending downwards and forwards to pubes, associated with frequent bilious acid vomiting and tossing about in agony without relief. (These are clinical symptoms, no doubt, but quite reliable.). Has been used in 3X potency as well as in the 200th. Its urine is quite characteristic; Urine of a saffron colour. Red (bloody) urine with brick-dust sediment after an attack of kidney pain.

Pariera: Nephralgia. Bruised pain in kidneys. Violent pains in bladder and at times in back; left testicle is painfully drawn up; frequently pains extend to thighs and even to toes and soles of feet (on attempting to pass water). Urine smells of ammonia. (Berberis has pains in back with extend to hips and its urine does not smell of ammonia.)

Pulmb: Kidney affection with albumen and sugar in urine. Colic with abdomen actually retracted (becomes concave). Kidney contracted (Aur-Mur., Nit-ac., Phos.). Rapid emaciation. Excessive debility. Constipation.

Arnic: Piercing pains as if a knife were being plunged into the region of kidneys; violent tenesmus of bladder. Chilly and inclined to vomit.

Helleb: Urine black or like coffee ground sediment; aluminous. Dropsy of chest, of abdomen. Frequent urging to urinate with scanty discharge.

Lyco: Nephralgia, pain along ureters into bladder, *esp.* right side. *A very severe pain is felt every time before urination, causing the patient cry out, pain ceasing as soon as urine begins to flow. *Red, sandy sediment in urine.

Phos: When kidney affections are associated with pneumonia, malignant pulmonary catarrh, or suppuration of bones. Copious watery diarrhoea (Chronic). Constant dull pain in region of right kidney: Can-ind. Pain in kidney when laughing: Can-ind. Throbbing in kidney region: Hepar.

LACTATION DERANGEMENTS

Therapeutics Leading Indications

Bryon: To dry up involuntary and profuse flow of milk, Bryon. 3X (Four to eight doses, four doses being required per day) is remarkably efficacious.

Calc-c: Involuntary flow of milk (galactorrhoea). Too profuse flow, with hectic. Too profuse, weakening. Scanty flow, mammae small. Milk tastes disagreeable, nauseating; child will not nurse and cries much.

Lac-d: Diminished secretion of milk in nursing women. It has the reputation of bringing back the milk in form 12 to 24 hours.

Merc-s: Milk scanty, spoiled, baby refuses to nurse. Deficiency of milk due to depressing sadness of mother: Agnus-c. Milk mixed with blood: Apis, Ipec., Phos. Milk mixed with pus: Cham. Flow of milk which curdles up speedily; Borax. Milk thin and of salty taste: Carb-an. Suppression of milk from exposure to cold and damp air: Dulc. Loss of milk without any other symptom any apparent causes: Urt-u. Milk runs out in nursing women: Calc-c., Cham., Phos., Rhus-t. Suppressed secretion of milk: Bell., Bryon., Calc-c., Caust., Dule., Puls. Suppressed from cold: Bryon., Dulc. Milk will not flow: Secale.

LEPROSY

Therapeutics Leading Indications

Arsen: Inflamed spots, chiefly in head, face, and neck. Small red pimples, which increase and change into gnawing ulcers, covered with a scurf. Spreads somewhat like ringworm, parts covered with silvery scales.

Carb-an: Erysipelatous inflammation. Swellings and burning pains. Foul discharges; burning, blueness. Anaemic, broken-down constitution.

Carb-ac: An excellent remedy for leprosy. Discharges offensive. Offensive odour from skin.

Graph: With humid eruptions. Deformity and thickness of nails. Obstinate dryness of skin and absence of perspiration.

Kali-od: When there is diffused soreness or sensitiveness over parts affected. Offensive odour in mouth. Frothy expectation. Worse from heat; aversion to heat.

Lach: Putremation of Flesh, which becomes detached from bones and falls off.

Nit-ac: Ulceration with cracks; very offensive odour from affected parts; sticking or pricking pains.

Secale: Skin of affected parts shriveled, dry and harsh. Gangrenous; ulcers black. Very offensive. Worse from warmth.

LEUCORRHOEA, WHITES

Characterized by secretion of mucus from vagina generally of a whitish colour origination in mucous of the vagina or the cavity of uterus, causes being numerous.

Therapeutics Leading Indications

Alumin: *Acrid and profuse, running down to heel (Syph.). Transparent, ropy and tenacious mucus. Worse during daytime and relieved by cold applications.

Amm-c: Very acrid, burning and water discharge; excoriating vulva.

Borax: Discharge like the white of an egg (Amm-m., Borax, Calc-o., Mezer.). With sensation as if warm water were flowing down.

Calc-c: In infants and before puberty. Discharge like milk and itching and burning; worse immediately before menses; too early and profuse menstruation; feet cold and damp. Corrosive leucorrhoea in young children.

Graph: Discharge very thin, watery white mucus, occurring. *It gushes day and night; often acrid and excoriating; great weakness in small of back when walking or sitting; before and after menses (before, sepia; after, Kros.).

Hydras. Ropy, thick, yellow, viscid; hanging from as in long strings (Kali-bi); great weakness; constipation; Pruritis.

Kreos: Putrid leucorrhoea which causes swelling and corrodes the parts, and there is itching as well as biting externally; leucorrhoea is exhausting; it may be milky, whey-like or yellow. Also corrosive, offensive leucorrhoea, causing redness and itching of vulva; of a yellow colour, staining linen yellow and stiffening like starch, with great weakness in legs; or white, having the adour of green corn with pain in small of back. Kreos. Leucorrhoea is worse between periods (Bavis., Borax) and is pronounced when standing and walking, hardly any when sitting or lying down.

Merc-s: Acrid, burning, itching with rawness; most troublesome at night; greenish discharge, itching or genitals worse from contact of urine which must be washed off (Sulph.). History of gonorrhoea; of syphilis.

Nit-ac: Mucus fetid, corrosive; fated discharge of a reddish brown colour; pricking pains. It has also ropy mucus like that of Kaki-bi. Itching. Swelling in burning of vulva and vegina. Excrescences on neck of uterus.

Puls: Discharge thick like cream or milky; thick yellowish and bland like all puls. Discharges. But sometimes corrosive and burning with itching of parts. Thick, white mucus; discharge taking place immediately before, during and after menstruation. Leucorrhoea in young girls who have not yet menstruated.

Sepia: Discharge like milk, only in daytime; with soreness of pudenda. Cheesy or curd-like discharge, which is horribly offensive. Ball-like (and heavy) sensation in vagina and uterus, associated with leucorrhoea and uterine troubles. It has also thick, creamy discharge. Discharge may be either bland or excoriating, but had smelling and pronounced before menses. Of gonorroeal origin.

Sulph: Profuse, yellowish, corrosive. Inveterate, chronic leucorrhoea with discharge of all kids (mild, excoriating etc.) and colours.

Aesc: When associated with more or less constant backache affecting.

Amm-m: Like white of an egg, preceded by pinching or griping pain about navel. May be brown, slimy, and painless or proceeded by pinching pains about navel discharged after making water. Two guiding concomitant symptoms are: (1) Violent pain in small of back *esp*. at night. (2) Inflation of belly. Arsenic—Profuse, thick, yellow, corroding, thin whitish; offensive discharge instead of menses; feeble weakly women.

China: Leucorrhoea instead of or preceding menses with painful pressing towards groins and Anus; bloody discharge with occasional discharge of black clots; fetid, purulent matter with troublesome itching in inner parts.

Carb-an: Burning and acrid; watery, offensive, staining line yellow; indurations and ulceration of the neck of uterus (Con.).

Carb-v: Thin and profuse, only in the morning on rising, not through day; milky; excoriating; soreness and rawness in pudenda.

Conium: Leucorrhoea, ten days after menses (Bar, Bov.); acrid; bloody; milky; profuse; thick; intermits. Indurations and ulceration of neck of uterus. In old maids.

Kali-c: Yellow, corrosive; pain in small of back, as if it would break.

Lill: Bright yellow, acrid excoriating, staining linen brown; "with severe bearing down in uterine region, worse afternoon till midnight, then better till next afternoon, when same symptoms return, ameliorated by sitting or lying down or by pressing with hands upon vulva."

Nux-v: Fetid, staining linen yellow; pressure towards genital organs, *esp.* towards morning; after allopathic drugging.

LIVER, AFFECTIONS OF (L. CIRRHOSIS)

Therapeutics Leading Indications

Acon: Pain in hepatic region hindering deep breathing (Bryon., lodi). Inflammation and sensation of soreness in liver. Hot, tense feeling in liver. Intolerable pains.

Arsen: Region of liver bloated, with violent burning pains. Vomiting of brownish or blackish substances. Black stools.

Bell: Acute pain in region of liver, worse from pressure, breathing, coughing, lying on right side, *jarring. *Tenderness of whole abdomen aggravated by least jar.

Bryon: Sharp stitching pains worse from motion and better from lying on right side. Pain under right shoulder-blade. Bitter taste in mouth. Liver enlarged. Lips parched and dry; great thirst.

Cardus: Liver region sensitive to pressure; liver enlarged in a transverse direction (Chel. More vertical). Liver and spleen both very enlarged so that they seem to fill the abdomen. Pressure, tension, and stitches in liver on lying on left side. Chronic liver diseases affecting lunges and causing vomiting of blood from lungs. Jaundice.

Chel: Liver enlarged; pain in hepatic region, better from eating. Abdomen distended and sensitive to pressure. Tenderness of liver to touch. Nausea and vomiting all the time. Constant tormenting urging in anus, but not better from drinking very hot water. Chronic diarrhoeas with liver troubles.

China: Pain in hepatic region as from subcutaneous ulceration. Liver swollen and hard, with tympanetic distention of abdomen. Where there is a history of loss of animal fluid.

Iodi: Swelling and hypertrophy of liver. Region of liver painful to pressure of touch. A low cache tic condition with profound debility and great emaciation.

Kali-c: Stitching pains in region of liver, not necessarily aggravated from motion, as in the case of Bryon. Burning pain, abscess has formed and suppuration has set in.

Lach: Generally called for after Bell. And Merc-s. in many cases of inflamation of liver. Patient cannot bear tight clothes around the waist. Enlarged liver of drunkards, with inflammation an abscess of liver. Pain as if something had lodged in right side of abdomen with stinging. When abscess in formed, Lach. is indicated by tenderness on pressure, intolerance to even pressure of clothing, abdomen being so sensitive to pressure. (Lyco. has also sensitiveness to pressure, but it is only after a meal, but in Lach., case, the sensitiveness is there all the time). Constant tormenting urging in the anus, but not after stool. After ague. After syphilis.

Lyco: A great anti-psoric remedy for liver affections. Its action on liver is very strong and deep. Pain in liver is dull and aching. Cannot bear the pressure of clothes about waist after a meal. Tension around region of liver, cannot stand or stretch upright. Distress in stomach immediately after eating. Fermentation in abdomen with loud rumbling, croaking, *esp*. in lower abdomen. Constipation. Violent hunger but a little quantity of food fills him up.

Nat-s: Soreness of liver to touch, to jars, with sharp stitching pains. Liver is engorged. Symptoms worse in wet weather.

Nit-ac: Useful in chronic enlargement of liver. Liver enormously large. Clay-coloured stool. Jaundice. Food odour from mouth profuse flow of saliva from mouth. Excessive weakness. Long-lasting cases of intermittent fever, with general cachexia and involved liver.

Podo: Indicated in chronic congestion and torpedity of liver, which is swollen and sensitive. Tongue coated yellow or white; dull headache; jaundice, face and eye yellow; bad state in the mouth. Constipation with clay-coloured stool, or loose watery stools, offensive, profound and gushing.

Chion: Has powerful action of liver. Hypertrophy of liver. "obstructed liver in malarias districts." Liver region sore to touch. Pain in liver and back. Liver enormously enlarged; constipation with clay-colours stool, bitter eructation's, bilious vomiting; sore aching on whole body; jaundice and high coloured urine. (3X or mother tincture are generally used. Three or four doses per day in watery solution are to be given.).

Ferr-ars: Enlarged liver and spleen with fever, 6th potency may be used. Twice daily for a few days and then to repeat with occasional stoppages.

Ferr-iod: Enlarged spleen and liver but no fever (6th potency.). To be repeated as in the case of Ferr-ars. Feels as if she had eaten too much, with a sort upward pressure. Costiveness. Suited to sacrofulous subjects and those persons who had relaxed fiber.

LOCHIAL DISCHARGE, DERANGEMENT IN

The vaginal discharges after confinement are called lochia. For the first few days of delivery, they are red, after three or four days they become pale and about the tenth day the colour becomes yellowish or yellowish white and, as a rule, cease altogether after a fortnight, although they may continue for several weeks.

Therapeutics Leading Indication

Aco: Suppresed lochia; fever with dry, hot skin and thirst.

Arsenic: A dose or two may be given.

Bapt: Lochia offensive. Feeling hot flushed face. Sensitive to slightest jar, which is unbearable; sleepy but cannot sleep.

Bryon: Sappression of lochia with splitting headache. Lips, mouth dry, with great thirst.

Dulk: Suppression of lochia from cold or dampness.

Kreos: Lochia very offensive; excoriating; black clots. mixed with water.

Secale: Lochia thin offensive; dark or black. Lochia suppressed, fever and enflmation of uterus.

LOCOMOTOR ATAXA

Wasting of spinal marrow resulting in disturbance in the co-ordination or motions.

Therapeutics Leading Indications

Alumin: Unable to walk except with eyes open and in daytime; staggers when closing eyes and when walking in dark. Feels as if he were walking on cushions. Formication or sensation as from creeping of ants in back and legs. Sensation as if there were cobeb on face, or as though the white of an egg were dried on it.

Arg-n: Great weakness of lower extremities with trembling. Staggers in dark or when walking with eye closed. Pain in small of back, severe when rising, but rather relieved by walking. Legs feel as if made of wood, with insensibility to touch. Emaciation of legs with paralytic weakness.

Phos: Burning along spine with much tingling and formication along spine and in affected extremities. Weakness and trembling of limbs, as if paralyzed. When walking makes missteps from weakness. Formication and tearing pains in legs.

Plumb: Advanced cases when there is wasting of paralyzed parts. Total loss of co-ordination. Extension of legs difficult or impossible, while flexion of legs sound. Loss of sexual desire or complete impotence.

Secale: "Absence of knee-jerk; fulgurating pains." "Shuffling gait as if feet were dragged along." "Difficult staggering gait, even complete inability to walk, not for want of power but on account of a peculiar unfitness to perform light movements with limbs and hands." Feeling as if walking on velvet. Formication, crawling and tingling in limbs.

Caust: Vertigo with tenancy to fall either forward or sideways and constant feeling of anxiety and weakness of head. Faint-like weakness with sinking of strength, with trembling.

Gels: Useful in fresh cases. Fatigue of lower limbs after slight exercise. Loss of muscular power in legs; they will not obey the will; staggering.

Kali-br: Nervous, busy, must keep oneself constantly occupied; hands and fingers in constant motions; fidgety hands. Inco-ordination of the muscles; nervous weakness. Memory almost lost; even forgets how to talk. Drowsiness.

Nux-v: When due to sexual excess. Lower limbs constantly trembling; fluttering of heart. Unsteady gait. Drags limbs in walking.

Physos: Great prostration of muscular system; constant inclination of sigh; staggering gait; tenderness of spine; muscles of back rigid. Muscles will not obey the will. Attacks of overpowering sleepiness. On walking, feeling of unsteadiness for legs downwards, so that he must look to see where he puts his feet.

Zinc: Lowered vitality. Numbness; Tingling; and Formication. Fidgety feet. Burning along whole length of spine. Backache markedly aggravated from sitting; better from walking about. (Nux-v. and Cham. Should not be used either before or after Zinc.)

LUMBAGO, BACKACHE

Rheumatic pain affecting the muscles of the lions is called lumbago. The pain comes on suddenly and generally lasts for a few days.

Lumbago

Calc-f: Lumbago worse after rest and on beginning in move, but relived by continued motion. Relieved by warmth. In lumbago arising from strains when Rhus-t proves ineffective. Calc-f. follows Rhus-t. well in chronic cases (to which it is similar).

Nux-v: "Lumbago, *esp.*, with constipation and weakness stiffness across loins; cannot turn in bed."

Rhus-t: Pain relieved by continued motion. Indicated is the beginning of lumbago, whether the patient is better from motion or not. Caused by wet damp weather or sudden cold.

Ant-t: Violent pain in lower part of back; slightest effort to move causes retching and cold, clammy sweat.

Act-t: Rheumatic pains in muscles of neck and back. Violent aching in back, sometimes extending down thigh.

Arnic: When caused by severe exertion. Worse slightest motion, *esp.*, when lying or getting warm bed.

Bell: Intensely painful sensation of cramps in small of back; can sit only for a short time and while sitting becomes stiff and unable to rise again for pain.

Bryon: Painful stiffness in small of back which do not allow walking or sitting upright. Stitching, tearing pains, worse from slightest motion. Dull aching in lamb muscles.

Coni: Cannot turn over in bed without being dizzy.

Ferr-m: Lumbago all night, goes off when rising.

Mag-p: Pains in back sharp. Shooting, boring and intermittent; better from warmth.

Ruta: Worse in morning before rising (Petrol); better after rising, Coccyx painful on sitting. Pain on back obstructing every movement.

Secale: Sudden 'catch' or 'kink' in the back. Worse from exertion or strain upon spine.

Backache

Arnica: When caused by severe exertion. Worse when in motion, *esp.*, when aggravated by walking or stooping. This symptom may be in connection with piles, leucorrhoea, displacement of uterus etc.

Cobalt: Back worse when sitting (Puls., Rhus-t., Zinc.). After or going off when rising up, walking or lying or lying down;. When caused by sexual excesses. Backache with seminal emissions.

Coni: See Lumbago. Very useful when backache is to bruises and shocks to the spine.

Kali-c: Backache while walking; feels as if they must give up and lie down; as a result of anaemia or after confinement, abortion, metrorrhagia etc. Sharp pains in back at 3 a.m., compelling one to get up and walk about. Intense pain in back for half an hour or more after every time she ate.

Nux-v: Backache generally worse at night while lying in bed; the patient must sit up to turn over. Pain is often in connection with pile as in the case of Aesc. caused by masturbation.

Puls: Pains in sacrum and back, as from long stooping or from a sprain. Better from rest and sleep. Backache relieved by slow motion. Chilliness (from suppressed menstruation).

Rhus-t: Rheumatic pains between scapulae, better from warmth, worse from cold. Stiffness and aching or bruised pains in small of back, when sitting still or when lying, better from motion or when laying on something hard (Nat-m.).

Zinc: spinal irritation, great prostration. Backache much aggravated by sitting, relieved by walking about (Cobalt, Puls., Rhus-t.). Burning along spine.

Bar-c: Stiffness and tension in small of back, aggravated in the evening to such an extent that one can hard rise up from chair and bend backwards. Cold feet.

Bryon: Painful stiffness in small of back compelling him to walk and sit crookedly. Wares from slight motion (Bryon. failing give Lyco. for this characteristic modality.)

Coccul: *Spinal weakness. Paralytic pain in small back, with spasmodic drawing across hips, prevents walking with anxiety and fear.

Guaiac: Stiffness of one side of back (usually of left side), from neck to small of back and sacrum, with intolerable pain on slightest motion or turning the part, noticed on touch or during rest.

Nat-m: Backache and spinal irritation, relieved by lying in something hard. Aggravation while lying down, *esp.* in morning. Caused by sexual excesses.

Physos: Stiffness and pain all down spine, muscles of back rigid. Great sense of fatigue and weariness. Irresistible desire to sleep.

Sepia: Pain in back and small of back, particularly with stiffness; relieved by walking (Rhus-t.), by pressing back against something hard.

MASTITIS

Inflammation of the breast is called mastitis.

Therapeutics Leading Indications

Apis: Burning, stinging pain in breast; swelling and hardness; great sensitiveness to touch: relief from cold applications. Erysipelatius inflammation.

Bell: Incipient stage of mammary abscess; breasts hard, swollen, feel heavy (Bryon.). Inflammation with red streaks running in radii; throbbing pain, burning heat; stitching pains appearing and disappearing suddenly. Aggravation form least jar. Characteristic fever (see Fever, simple).

Bryon: In threatening mammary abscess; stony heaviness of breast, *stitching pains worse from slightest motion. Swelling and hardness but little or no redness. Nausea and faintness.

Hepar: When suppuration is threatening. It may prevent it (use high potency, say 200th) or when suppuration in inevitable or when scanty discharge of pus is taking place, it will hasten the process of suppuration, for which purpose use a low potency, say 3X or 6, although even the 200th potency can well be used with advantage as it hastens suppuration admirably, as verified in my practice. Indications are: Extreme sensitiveness to touch and sharp splinter-like pains.

Merc-s: Often called for after Bell., when in spite of that remedy pus begins to form, characteristic indications being: chilliness transient, creeping; *profuse sweat without relief. (When there is little or no pus, a high potency will often prevent suppuration, but when much pus is formed, a low potency will hasten the process.)

Phyt: *Breast very hard, swollen, hot. Burning and painful *esp.* indicated when from the beginning of mastitis, hardness is very apparent. From the onset there is a tendency to that is called "caked breast" (for which it is almost a specific). Often indicated after Bryon.

Silic: Fistulous opening discharging thin, fetid, watery pus and slow to heal. Absorbs indurations left after suppuration.

MASTURBATION

The gratifying of sexual desire by artificial means. The effects are pernicious.

Therapeutics Leading Indications

Calc-c: One of the greatest remedies often called for after self-abuse. (Two other great remedies are Nax-v. and Sulph.). Great depression of spirits, fatigue with nervous weakness. Palpitation of heart and confusion of ideas. Sexual power diminished. Cold feet at night in bed. Decisively weak after a short walk.

China: Relieves weakness from masturbation. Symptoms after long-continued masturbation: Pale, sickly expression; face pale and sallow; eyes sunken and surrounded by blue and dark margins;

throbbing headache; perspiration very profuse and debilitating, *esp*. at night; sweat easily on least excretion.

Nux-v: Emissions, *esp*. towards morning with fatigue on waking. Digestion impaired. Feels fatigued or un refreshed in morning on waking.

Staph: Long-standing cases. Face sunken; guilty, abashed facial expression; loss of memory, sadness; hypochondrias is; nocturnal emissions; backache; weak legs; lusterless eyes; hair falls out; general weakness; sexual organs relaxed; tendency to take cold easily.

Sulph: It is apt toward off the tendency to this bad habit (a-dose of Calc-c. 30 may be given a fortnight after a dose sulph. 30 has been administered.). Sexual organs relaxed and cold. Frequent pollutions. Pain in back; dejection; heat on vertex.

Kali-br: Bad effects of sexual excesses: unsteady gait; cannot stand erect, legs weak; inco-ordination of muscles; confused; nervous; impotant. Drowsiness. Vision dim, almost gone. Intellectual faculties greatly impaired. *Memory absolutely lost; even forgets how to talk. Absent minded. In writing omits words or part of words.

Phos: When the patient suffers from painless, debilating chronic diarrhoea. Weakness and weariness; nervous debility and trembling. Pain in chest. Distressed by the culpability of his indulgence.

Phos-ac: Subdues uncontrollable desire for self-abuse in young boys; bad effects of pre-pubic masturbation. Much distressed by the culpability of the act. Great physical and mental weakness form sexual excesses. Weak feeling in chest from talking, Grows too fast and too tall. Discharge of prostatic fluid during stool.

Puls: Masturbation practiced by females resulting in leucorrhoea or hysterical affections.

MEASLES

A contagious, eruptive fever, chiefly affecting children and attended with sneezing, running of nose, redness and watering of eyes, hard cough, bronchial affections, and even pneumonic symptoms.

Therapeutics Leading Indications

Acon: Often indicated in the beginning of an attack. Fever with quick, full pulse; *dry hot skin with restlessness. Dry, hacking and even croupy caugh.

Bell: In the beginning when there is fever with moist skin, red eyes, flushed face, sleepy but cannot sleep; dry cough with tickling in larynx; head hot, legs cold; jerking of limbs during sleep; abdomen bloated.

Bryon: When eruptions are slow to appear and there is hard, dry, painful cough; little or no expectoration; constipation; dry lips and tongue with great thirst. Also when eruptions suddenly disappear and brain symptoms develop. Stitching pains in chest.

Gels: In the beginning (Generally after Acon.). Fever with drowsiness; "a feeling of great weight and tiredness in the entire body and limbs"; watery discharge from nose, excoriating wings of nose and upper lips; hard, barking and croupy cough with hoarseness; suffused face. Also when eruptions turn livid and brain symptoms develop.

Ipec: Eruptions slow to appear with difficulty in breathing; much nausea and vomiting; rattling or wheezing of phlegm in chest.

Puls: Not indicated in the beginning and never to be given in course of fever at the commencement. Coryza and profuse lachrymation; cough dry at night and loose a daytime. There may be earache. Fever in late stages with dry lips and no thirst. Eruptions slow in coming out or when fully out have a dark appearance. Dry lips which the patient constantly licks with tongue, but no thirst. Discharge from nose thick yellow. Chronic loose cough after measles.

Apis: Confluent eruptions and oedematous swelling of skin; cough with soreness of chest as from a bruise; difficulty in breathing with inability to remain in warm room.

Arsenic: In severe cases with typhoid symptoms; sudden disappearance of eruptions; face bloated; great anguish and fear of death; symptoms worse after midnight.

Zinc: When the child is too weak to develop the erptions; child cries out in sleep and awakes from terrified.

MENINGITIS

Inflammation of brain substance is called Encephala of its membranes, Meningitis. It is very difficult to distinguish one from the other. Such discrimination is, however, essential to homoeopathic treatment.

Meningitis is, in great majority of cases, association with diseases like Typhoid fever, Measles, Pneumonia etc. The actual disease suddenly manifests itself convulsion or fever with pain in head, rush of blood to the head, vomiting etc.

Therapeutics Leading Indications

Acon: In the first stage of inflammation. Skin hot, high fever, red face, unquenchable thirst, quick restlessness, anxiety and fear, When caused by exposure too.

Apis: Fidgetiness; sudden shrill cry in sleep. Inflammation caused by suppressed or undeveloped eruption. Burning, stinging pain. Urine suppressed or frequent, pain and scanty.

Bell: Face red, violent throbbing in head, red eyes. Great sensitiveness to light and noise. Violent headache sudden starting from sleep.

Bryon: When caused by suppressed eruptions. Dark red, lips dry and parched, great thirst for large quantity of water at long intervals. Wants to keep perfectly still so the leas motion makes him worse.

Canth: Inflammation of brain violent anger amazing to paroxysms of rage, with cries, barking liked biting at any one approaching him. Burning pain. Slightest touch aggravates pain. Irritation of bladder; scalds him.

Cicu: From concussions of brain or suppressed lions. Violent convulsions with frightful distortions of and whole body with loss of consciousness; rolling of head from side to side.

MENORRHAGIA, METRORRHAGIA

Menorrhagia is meant profuse menstruation.

Therapeutics Leading Indications

Aconite: Menses too early and profuse; profuse discharge in night red blood which feels hot as it passes, throbbing pain; great bearing down as if everything would protrude vulva.

Cal-c: Menses too early, too profuse., too long-lasting; exertion or least excitement causes return of menses due to coldness. *sensations as if she had on cold, damp place.

Kreoso: Menses too early, profuse and lasting too long; flow intermits, at times almost ceases and then comes again; flow worse from or on lying down, better of ceasing sitting and walking about. Discharge offensive. Uterus hemorrhage with the same symptoms.

Nux-v: Menses too early, too profuse, too long last irregular, never at right time. After continuing for several stops and then flows again.

Puls: Hemorrhage ceases for a little while and recommences with redoubled force. Blood may be dark mixed with coagulated lumps.

Sabin: Menses to early, too profuse and also long lasting; flow partly fluid, partly clotted (Plat., Ferr flow in paroxysms; colic and labour-like pains; pain back to pubes.)

Secale: Best adapted to thin, scrawny women. Dark fluid, flow may come to gushes and produce strong bearing down pains. Continuous, bloody, discharge between two periods are rather prolonged so that it is practically speaking a continuous flow. Thin, black, horribly offensive flow. Great debility. Or hemorrhage of the aforesaid character after abortion.

MENTAL DERANGEMENT

Therapeutics Leading Indications

Calc-c: Fears that when will lose her reason or understanding, and that the people would observe her mental confusions.

Canth: Acute mania of a sexual type, amorous frez Sexual appetite is aroused to be point of mania.*burning in urethra.

Coni: Suited to old maids, widows, and bachelors, when ailments arise from ungratified sexual desire.

Hepar: Attacks of mania with quick, hasty speech irritability from slightest cause.

Hyos: Very suspicious. Fear of being poisoned. Mania characterized by immodestly, will not remain cover exposes genital organs. Mutters absurd things to himself Mania with buffoonery and ridiculous gesture.

Ignat: Slightest contradiction excites her anger, make one angry with oneself. Inward grief from disappointing love or mortification. *Full of suppressed grief; with the drawn sighs.

Kali-bar: Gets fidgety, must do something, off above (Tarant.). "Constantly busy in tying his shoes, fumble his pockets, picking threads etc."

Lach: Great loquacity; wants to talk all the time; Jump from one subject to another; one word often leads into and story, or into the midst of another story. Thinks she is under superhuman power. Sense as to time of the day is dream.

Nat-m: Sad and depressed; consolation aggravates. Hysterical girls who fall in love with persons, where the relationship is offensive to polite ear.

Nat-s: Loathing of life, suicidal impulses, *great restrain being necessary to avoid bodily harm.

Puls: Can hardly narrate her symptoms without weeping. *She weeps at everything whether it is joyful or sorrowful.

Sepia: Hysterical diathesis. *Great sadness with tears.

Staph: Violent outbursts of passion. Shy of the opposite sex.

Stram: *Praying and singing devoutly, beseeching, entreating. Talking continually and foolishly. Ungovernable desire to bite, to strike, or to kill. (Use the 30th potency.).

Sulph: Fears she will not be saved. Have insane ideas. Everything looks pretty which the patient takes a fancy to, even sags rags beautiful.

Tarant: Must be doing something all the time. Constant involuntary movements to legs, arms, trunk; unable to do anything. Extreme sexual excitement. Music has exciting effects at first, but later in relieves symptoms.

METRITIS

It means inflammation of uterus.

Therapeutics Leading Indications

Arsen: *Esp*. In childhood; from great losses of blood from uterus.

Bell: After abortion (Sabin.). Sensitiveness to least jar.

Canth: Swelling of neck of uterus; burning; tenderness; suppuration.

Hepar: With throbbing, and sensitiveness to slight pressure on pelvis region.

Hydras: Endo-metritis; aching pain in back, debility and digestive disorder.

Lac-c: With soreness and tenderness making every motion, position, and even breathing painful.

Sabi: After premature labor.

MISCARRIAGE, ABORTION

Expulsion of the product of conception during the first three months is termed abortion.. When the expulsion of the fetus takes place from this time to viability (state of the fetus when it is capable of living outside of the uterus), it is designated immature delivery or miscarriage. Expulsion from the period of viability the full term is called premature delivery.

Therapeutics Leading Indications

Acon: Threatened abortion from anger, *esp*. fright; fears that something terrible is going to happen to her; dizziness on rising from a recumbent position.

Arnic: Threatened abortion as a result of fall, blow, shock, concussion, particularly when blood comes out without pain. *Sore pain all over body as if from a bruise.

Bell: Severe bearing down. As if everything would protrude through vulva; pains come on suddenly and cease suddenly.

Caul: With severe pain in back and loins but uterine contraction feeble; slight flow. Habitual abortion from uterine a tony.

China: If hemorrhage continues after abortion and there is giddiness, drowsiness and fainting. Extremely useful in removing the after-effects of hemorrhage, heaviness in head, ringing in ears, coldness of extremities.

Helon: A "Uterine tonic". Useful in threatened abortion from atonics conditions, *esp.*, in habitual abortion.

Plumb: Tendency to abortion from non-development of ulcers Muscular fibers of ulcers do not develop proportionally as the fetus increases in size in uterus and consequent abortion.

Puls: *Flow ceases for a while, then returns with redouble forces; *this process of cessation and return is often repeated craves fresh air.

Rhus-t: When caused by strain or wrench. Pain work latter part of night and during rest; must change position for relief.

Sabin: Threatened miscarriage, *esp.* during third month with pain commencing in the small of back and going round and through the pubes. *Pain runs through from sacrum to pubes. Bright red, clotted flow of blood on Bright red blood, partly fluid and partly clotted increasing with every motion.

Secale: Prolonged bearing down, forcing pains: Copious flow of black liquid blood. Especially after miscarriage has taken place; thin, black, foul-smelling discharge; work for least motion. Great debility and extinct pulse.

Sulph: "Promotes expulsion of moles or blighted conceptions and cures the predisposition to abort in future conceptions.

Cinnamonum: Profuse flow of bright red blood (Bell., Ipec.); after a false step or strain in loins.

Gels: Pains may leave uterus and fly all over body Loss of muscular power. Nervous chills.

Homan: There is great soreness in the abdomen.

Ipec: Cutting pains around navel; profuse and continued flow of bright red blood; continual nausea.

MORNING SICKNESS

Characterized by nausea, vomiting, heartburn accompanying pregnancy. Consult the article on vomiting and nausea.

Therapeutics Leading Indications

Nit-ac: Nausea and gastric troubles relieved by moving about or riding a carriage. Strong-smelling urine.

Petrol: "Applicable to all gastric troubles of pregnant women." Incessant nausea and qualmishness in morning with accumulation of water in mouth; aversion to fat food or meat. Diarrhoea only during day time.

Sepia: Gone. Empty feeling in stomach, not relieved by eating. Constipation. Thought of food sickens her; nausea from smell of food; Nausea in morning, passing off after eating something.

Lac-ac: Nausea on awaking; better after eating. Constant nausea; persisting for days. Nausea and vomiting; water-brash relieved by breakfast.

Nux-v: Nausea, particularly when sickness is felt at the stomach. Nausea after eating; in morning. She feels that if she could only vomit, she would be much better.

Gossypium: Morning nausea and salivation. Inclination to vomit before breakfast, Faintness, cannot rise from bed. Morning sickness during early months.

Iris: Nausea which may be protracted; vomiting with burning in mouth, throat and gullet. Vomiting is bilious, watery, acrid.

Vomiting with deathly nausea: Tabac. Vomiting of sweetish water before breakfast; Kreos. More nausea then vomiting: Ipec. Long continued vomiting, cannot retain food in stomach: Kali-bi.

MUMPS, PAROTITIS

Inflammation of the parotid gland, the largest pair of the salivary glands under the ear and near the angle of the lower jaw.

Therapeutics Leading Indications

Bar-c: In the case of scrofulous person, when other glands are swollen at the same time; when glands grow. Glands around ears painful and swollen. Affects right ear. And right parotid most.

Bell: Swelling bright red and hot, *esp.*, on right side, or when swelling suddenly disappears, resulting in brain troubles, such as delirium, unconsciousness etc. Stitches extend into ears.

Bryon: When swelling suddenly disappears and alarming brain symptoms ensue.

Merc-s: Swelling is pale; jaws are stiff; tongue flabby takes the imprint of teeth. Salivary glands swollen and painful. Profuse salivation.

Phyto: Parotid and sub-maxillary glands swollen. Violent cases with difficulty swallowing. Fetid breath.

Rhus-t: Swelling and inflammation of parotids with fever; swelling is dark red; left side particularly affected; or left side is more affected than right. Suppuration of parotids. Inflammation has an erysipelatous character. *N.B.* Rhus-t.. Seems to be a great weapon in our hands. In a case I was led to the selection of the remedy, simply because of the fact that the patient could with difficulty open the mouth, but persistent attempt to open the mouth had the effect of mitigating pain and stiffness. The case was radically cured with Rhus-t.

Arsen: Mumps associated with fever, measles. Small-pox. (Of a malignant type. Paroxysmal and unbearable pain. (Author) Anxious restlessness.

Carb-v: When swelling does not subside, but grows harder. Hoarseness.

Cistus: Swelling and indurations of parotid and neck glands in scrofulous subjects who are sensitive to cold air. Stitching pains. Worse from bathing.

Crotal: Of a malignant type, associated with neuralgia around affected parts. (Author). Right side *esp*. affected.

Lach: Malignant; swelling purplish.

NAILS, AFFECTIONS OF

Therapeutics Leading Indications

Ant-c: Nails discolored and deformed. Nails do not grow rapidly, Split nails, growing cracked and thick. This may occur after mechanical injury. Split hoops in the case of horses (Farrington).

Fluor-ac: Nails grow rapidly; nails brittle, crumble and have longitudinal furrow.

Graph: Nails grow thick, cracked, out of shape; nails brittle, crumbling. Painful, sore.

Hyper: Injuries to fingers, toes and matrices of nails.

Silic: Deep-seated inflammation; violent pain deep in finger; worse in warm bed; opening with a surrounding of proud flesh. Crippled nails on fingers and toes. Offensive foot-sweat. In growing toe-nails.

Thuja: "Finger-nails distorted, crumbling, soft, distorted; in growing toe-nails."

NERVOUSNESS

Therapeutics Leading Indications

Acon: Mental restlessness: anxiety; feels he will die.

Arnic: Great sensitiveness of mind with anxiety and restlessness. Tendency to be frightened.

Arg-n: Always in a hurry but accomplished nothing.

Well: Nervous anxiety, restlessness, desire to escape. Disinclination to talk or very fast talking.

Cham: Mental excitement with strong tendency to be frightened. Peevish, Quarrelsome.

Gels: Dread of death: utter lack of courage. Dread of falling. State fright. Nervous dread of appearing in public (Arg-n.). The anticipation of any unusual ordeal brings on dirrhoea. Dirrhoea on preparing for churck, theatre, or to meet an engagement. Fears that unless on the move heart will cease beating. Nervous exhaustion, wants to lie down and rest.

Lyco: Afraid to be alone. "Dreads lest something will happen, lest he will forget something." Dread of appearing in the public, as at times, such is the case with professional men, who, however, after the task is under taken, accomplish it with smoothness. (This is like Silicia.).

Mag-c: "Worn-out women" with nervousness from excess of cares and worries of life. Exhausted nerves. Sad mood with disposition to talk.

Mag-p: Dullness and inability to think clearly: highly nervous (the patient is usually thin, emaciated). Can think and study more clearly after a few doses of Mag-p.

Merc-s: Great nervousness (constantly changing from place to place), with fear of losing the reason. Hurried and rapid speech.

Syph: Very nervous, walks much of the time; weeps without cause. Afraid of night.

NEURALGIA

Pain of a purely nervous character, recurring in paroxysms and is usually not attended with inflammation. For neuralgia affecting nerves of head, heart and nates to the knees and sometimes to the ankles, refer to the articles on Headache, Angina pectoris, and Sciatica.

Therapeutics Leading Indications

Acon: From exposure to dry, cold winds. Pains drive the patient almost to despair; tingling in affected parts numbness; pains worse at night, in evening.

Act-r: Neuralgia, sharp laminating, Electric-like pains in various parts, arising from uterine and ovarian irritations. In uterine region darting from side to side. Intend aching pains in eye-balls (Spig.); worse moving head or eyes, better lying down.

Arsen: Malarial neuralgias. Violent nocturnal pains exciting despair and fury. Burning with pains; relieved by heat.

Bell: pains come on suddenly, last a shorter or longer period and then disappear suddenly. Pains worse from motions slightest jar, light or noise; worse 2 to 6 p.m.; right side mostly affected.

Cham: Exceedingly sensitive to pain, so that least pain becomes unbearable. Pain causes hot perspiration about head and starts cries; very irritable, can hardly speak or answer clearly.

China: Neuralgia *esp.* of malarial origin, generally infra-orbital of either side; typical in their periodical return; worse from slightest touch or draught of cold air. Pains worse every other day (Arsen., Not-m.).

Coloc: Pains come on suddenly and after a while disappear as suddenly as they had come. *Sudden atrocious cramping pain, causing twisting, turning around to obtain relief, and crying out with pain. Relief from hard pressure. Its intense neuralgic pains are found in face ache, iritis, glaucoma, colic, sciatica, and ovaritis. (*N.B.*: Pressure gives relief to intense pain in the beginning, later, pressure may aggravate them. Intensity of pain may cause even fainting.)

Mag-p: Pains better from heat. Excruciating pains intermittent, spasmodic, lightning-like pains; worse from touch, cold air, pressure; better from external heat; exhausting. *Sudden paroxysms of pain extorting cries. *Crimpy pains are highly characteristic. Neuralgic every night shifting from place to place. Severe neuralgic pains in ears. Vesicle neuralgia after use of catheter. Right side mostly affected.

Spig: Sharp and very violent neuralgic pain affecting left eye; relieved by pressure. *Left-sided neuralgic head face and eye. Neuralgic pains come on and go with the sun, gradually increasing with the advance of the day, at its climax at soon, and then declining with sun. Pains, as a rule, press out.

Stan: Pains increase and decrease gradually. Pains at times so violent that the mind seems stunned and even the patient may faint.

Abrot: Neuralgia of head and stomach due to metastasis.

Clem: Drawing pains in testes and in spermatic cord, extending to groins and thighs.

Cup-ar: Neuralgia of abdominal viscera, or rather simply say, intense neuralgic pain in abdomen. Often excited by damp weather.

Hamam: Neuralgia of testicles (Ustilago).

Syph: Sharp pains here and there. Pains wonder about all over body. Pains affect parts in a straight line.

Thuja: Neuralgia of tea drinkers. Attacks of excruciation pain from right kidney downward: sar. Everyday at same hour: Cedr., Kali-bi. Neuralgia of coccyx; worse rising from a sitting posture; must sit still: Lach.

NIGHT-BLINDNESS

The patient sees well in bright light, but as soon as the intensity of light falls short of what he requires for his vision, cannot see the surrounding objects, be it light or candle-light.

Therapeutics Leading Indications

Bell: Can see nothing dusk; red or fiery spots before eyes; sees as coloured halo around the candle.

Lyco: Eyes get dazzled and irritated by candlelight in evening; Black spots floating before eyes.

Sulph. Night-blindness; sees a halo around a lamplight; cataract.

Puls. With menstrual disturbance, as eyes were lightly bound.

Lyc: Must stop work at 4 p.m.

NIGHTMARE

A frightful dream during which the patient feels pressure in the breast but cannot speak or move.

Therapeutics Leading Indications

Guaiac: Nightmare, when lying on back, waking with screams. Feels un refreshed on waking up. Frequent awaking with fright.

Kali-br: Nightmare, full of fearful dreams. Night terrors of children; they scream in their sleep an want to inding to the nurse (Hyos.).

Mezer: Wakes early (towards 2 or 3 a.m.) in consequence of nightmare.

Nit-ac: Sleep un refreshing. Many fantastical, anxious and frightful dreams. Shocks in body and jerking in limbs during sleep.

Nux-v: Caused by indulgence in alcoholic liqueurs of too high living. Awakes in fright from least noise.

Opium: Sleeps with eyes half-closed, with mouth vide open; deep snoring, rattling in throat. Cold sweat.

Puls: Nightmare caused by rich, fat food or meat. Sleepless first parts of night. Cries and moans in sleep.

Sulph: Dreams fantastic, frightful, horrible. Cries moans, snores, lies on back with arms above head.

OPHTHALMIA

Inflammation of the eye, *esp.* of the conjunctiva, being the lining of the eyelids and the external coat of the eyeball. May be catarrhal, scrofulous, rheumatic, gouty, syphilitic or of gonorrheal origin.

Incidentally, other ailments of the eye have also been dealt with in this article as will be observed on a study of the remedies.

Therapeutics Leading Indications

Acon: Ophthalmic following surgical operations, or resulting from a foreign body in the eye or any injury. From exposure to dry, cold winds, with great deal of heat, dryness and burning in eyes.

All-c: Profuse, non-excoriating lachrymator; copious watery, excoriating discharge from nose. Worse in evening and in warm room.

Apis: Conjunctiva red, puffy, chemotic: great relief of pain from cold water. Characteristic pain: burning, stinging, and sore. Great sensitiveness of eyes to light.

Rhus-t: Oedematous swelling of lids; hot gushing larchrymation. Formation of pus. Eyelids feel heavy and stiff. Pain worse at night, *esp*. after midnight. Warmth relieves.

Arg-n: Purulent ophthalmic: pus is thick, yellow, bland, and profuse. *Esp*. after the failure of Puls. or Mesc-s., or Merc-cor. Symptoms relieved by cold air or water. This modality is a gem. (Author). Worse from warmth. Complains to little or no trouble. Farrington says that when Arg-n. Ceases to act (or rather flag. as I would prefer to say), a dose of Puls. if interpolated, helps.

Arsen: Inflammation of eyes and lids, with *burning pain, worse after midnight, better from warm applications; *mental restlessness. Corrosive lachrymator. Oedematour eyelids.

Dulc: Inflammation of eyes from exposure to damp cold air.

Euph: Profuse excoriating lachrymator, with profuse bland crazy (reverse of All-c.). eyes agglutinated in morning. Ulceration of eye, developing thick, excoriates discharge. Little blisters on or near cornea. Pimples on the part of the cheek over which tears flow. Also: thick, purulent discharge, but this is also excoriating. Obscuration of vision causing frequent winking.

Hepar: With superlative tendency; throbbing in and around eye; great sensitiveness of affected parts to touch. Ulcer in cornea; intense photophobia; pains relieved by external warmth.

Hyper: Pain and irritation of eye being the result of injury or wounds, which might have occurred several years ago.

Kali-bi: Chronic indolent forms of ophthalmic affections, *esp*. syphilitic. May be scrofulous or synoptic. Secretion of a stringy character. Pus or secretion yellow. Yellow pus in acanthi. Lids agglutinated in morning.

Kreos: Inflammation of eyelid, in children or adults; discharge of hot, scalding tears in morning. Heat and burning in eyes: tears are acrid like salt water. "Eyes feel as if in woody smoke."

Marc-c: May be of catarrhal, scrofulous, syphilitic on gonorrheal origin. *Great violence of symptoms. Inflammation and swelling intense; burning, agonizing pain; intense photophobia. Profuse, excoriating lachrymation, making cheeks sore. Tearing pains around bones of eyes. Ulceration of cornea with tendency to perforation. Ophthalmic of inborn babies, with acrid discharges cause by syphilitic or gonorrheal leucorrhoea in mother.

Merc-s: Excessive sensitiveness of eyes to glare and heat of fire. Pains worse at night and in damp weather. Lids spasmodically closed. Lachrymation profuse, burning and excoriating.

Puls: Discharge thick, bland, yellow. Symptoms better in open air. Ophthalmic after measles. In newborn babies. Gonorrhoeal: *after sudden suppression of gonorrheal discharge. (Here the asterisk is mine.)

Staph: Inflammation and itching of margins of lid. Pains extend to teeth. Syphilitic iritis with bursting. Pain in eyeball, temple and side of face, worse from evening to morning and on using eyes by any light.

Coni: Scrofulous; great intolerance of light, without inflammation of eye. Complicated with glandular affection *esp.* around neck.

Graph: Lids thickened, particularly along edges, which are covered with scurf's and scales. Lids tend to crack a bleed. Eyelashes turn inwards and irritate the eye. Vesicles on cornea and on other parts of eye with profuse thin, acrid discharge.

Kali-c: Oedema of lids, particularly *bag-like swelling between upper eye lids and eyebrows.

Kali-s: Yellow discharge; worse from warmth and in evening better in open air. This yellow discharge may be water or pus-like. Yellow crusts on eyelids. Ophthalmic newborn babies with yellow discharge.

ORCHITIS

Inflammation of the Testis

Aconite: In the first stage of acute orchitis its action is something wonderful. Although our texts do not endorse, its action in painful gonorrheal orchitis is decisive. (My experience.) Orchitis cause by taking cold (Puls., Rhus tox.). Prescribe Aconite 3X first.

Clematis: Testicles indurate with bruised feeling. Swelling of the right half of scrotum and testes. Painful inflammation and swelling of testes. Testes as hard as stone.

Merc-sol: Testes hard and swollen, with shining redness of scrotum and dragging pain in testes and spermatic cords. Gonorrheal.

Nitric-acid: Inflammatory swelling of testes, with painful drawing of the spermatic cord, as far as side of abdomen. Frequent pollutions.

Nux-v: Inflammatory swelling of testes with painful sensitiveness to touch, hardness and retraction of testes.

Phytolacca: Orchitis with suppuration and fistulous ulcers.

Spong: Hard swelling of testes. Heat in testes, scrotum and cords. Chronic, worse at full moon. Maltreated orchitis. After suppressed gonorrhea.

OTORRHOEA

Discharge from ears, frequently due to suppuration in the middle ears.

Therapeutics Leading Indications

Arsen: Profuse, ichorous, cadaverously smelling discharge; voluptuous tickling and burning in ears. Intense pain.

Bar-m: Discharge smelling like rotten cheese, abscess behind ears. Parroted, *esp*. right swollen.

Calc-c: Discharge purulent, "of a sort of pappy of fatty appearance," "looking just like chewed up paper." Drum perforated by ulceration.

Caps: Chronic suppuration of ear. Painful swelling on the bone behind ear; pain worse from touch. Deep-seated swelling under ear; tearing pain deep in ear. Drumhead perforated, discharge of thick, yellow pus; itching deep in ear; burning in ears.

Cist: Discharge of watery, fated, offensive pus; swelling of parotid glands. The patient is very sensitive to cold air.

Hepar: Discharge of fetid pus from ears. Discharge smelling like old cheese. Heat, redness and itching in ear. Relief from hot applications.

Lyco: Offensive, chorus, purulent discharge from ear, without hardness of hearing. External meatus excoriated.

Merc-s: Purulent, offensive discharge from ears. Discharge of pus and blood (which is sometimes the case after an attack of small-pox). Ulceration of external ear. Inflammatory swelling of parotids. its action on the cellular tissues in deeper than that of Puls.

Puls: *Profuse, thick, yellow or yellowish green discharge from ears. It is bland and practically inoffensive. Better in open air and during day; worse at night, Otorrhoea alternating with difficult hearing.

Tell: Formation of pus in middle ear and perforation of drumhead. "Itching and swelling, with painful throbbing in external meatus; in three or four days, discharge of watery fluid, smelling like fish pickle, which cause vesicle wherever it touches; ear is blistered, as if oedematous; hearing impaired." Persistent, fetid body odour. Eczema behind ear.

Calc-p: Excoriating discharge from the ears. Complication with tuberculosis.

Caust: Offensive discharges, sometimes oozing of blood form ears; meatus swollen and excoriated; words and steps re-echo in ears.

Elaps: Offensive, yellow-greenish discharge; discharge of blood from ears, which may be black. Ear-wax black. Eruption behind ears with sticky secretions or crusty eruptions on ears and cheeks.

Kali-bi: Discharge of fetid, thick, yellow pus, which is mixed with *stringy mucus. Itching deep in ear.

ABSCESS OF MEATUS

This affection does not legitimately come under the category of Otorrhoea, but we would like to treat the same here.

An abscese of the meatus is very painful and has the tendency to recur. if the tendency to recurrence is not eradicated, the walls of the meatus as well as the drum become thickened, invariably causing impairment of hearing sooner or later.

In the beginning of inflammation, characterized by heat, redness and throbbing, give a few doses of Bell. 3X or 30 and later on, if required, a dose of Marc-s. 30, which often prevents suppuration, it is given in the beginning. But Merc-s. is especially indicated after suppuration has taken place, when it promotes discharge of pus.

After Bell., Hepar may be called for when there is great sensitiveness to touch of the affected parts and relief from warm application.

Pic-ac: Reputed to be almost a specific for small furuneles in exterior part of ear-hole. If given early it aborts the abscess; in advanced state, it ameliorates the conditions. Besides, it has the tendency to prevent recurrence of the disease.

Syph: Indicated in abscess in left ear, discharging a great quantity of pus (hereditary syphilis in children).

OVARIES, AFFECTIONS OF

Two oval bodies situated on each side of the womb, connected with the same by the broad ligaments are called ovaries. Inflammation of the ovary or its membrane, termed ovaritis, is caused by getting wet during menstruation, exposure to cold winds, sudden suppression of menses, gonorrhea etc.

Therapeutics Leading Indications

Acon: Overbites after exposure to dry, cold winds; after suppression of menses from being chilled or as a result of fright.

Apis: *Esp*. Affects right ovary (Bell.); ovary swollen and extremely sensitive to touch with *stinging burning pains; pain in right ovary with pain in left chest caused by shock of coughing; no thirst, scantly urine.

Arsen: *Esp*. affect right ovary; burning; lancinating pains, as of hot coals were burning in the part. Relieved by hot application, with restlessness; somewhat relieved by moving feet.

Bell: *Esp*. affects right ovary; throbbing pains; *pains appear and disappear suddenly; great bearing down with feeling as if everything would protrude from vulva; great tenderness, *cannot bear slightest jar; fever with sweat on covered parts.

Bryon: Stitching pains in ovaries on deep inspiration; worse from least motion; suppression of menses with bleeding of nose.

Canth: Much burning in ovarian region arresting breathing; or violent pinching pains with bearing down towards genitals; constant urging to urinate with painful discharge of a few drops of urine.

Coni: Chronic overitis; indurations and swelling of ovary after contusions with lancination pains; soreness and swelling of breast before menses; intermittent flow of urine.

Hamam: Overbitis after a blow. (Arnica); ovary swollen with a diffused agonizing soreness over whole abdomen; menses irregular and very painful; of gonorrheal origin.

Hepar: When suppuration is imminent (Lach., Merc-s.) or has occurred, frequent chill; throbbing pains; pricking pains. Sweats without relief. (May be associated with chronic gonorrhea.)

Iodi: Indurations and swelling of ovary (Coni.), with tendency of cancerous degeneration. pain commences in right ovary passing down broad ligament to uterus (Hammam). Chronic ovaritis (left) with thick, yellow, burning leucorrhoea better after eating (H.N. Martin). Great sensitiveness of right ovarian region during or after menses.

Lach: Has special affinity for ovaries. Called for in various ovaries ovarian ailments, such as, neuralgia, inflammation, suppuration, even tumors and cancer of one or both ovaries, but principally the left one. What is highly characteristic is when *the left ovary is attacked first, and then the right one. Pain in ovary (*esp.* the left), relieved by a discharge from uterus. "Shooting pains (left) extending from the left to the right ovarian region (Lit-t.). "Neuralgic pains (left ovary) with tenderness to pressure of the clothing." Inability to lie on right side, on account of sensation as if something were rolling over to that side. When pus has formed, it will promote the discharge (Haper, Merc-s.).

Arg-m: Bruised pain in left ovary and sensation at if the ovary growing very large.

Merc-s: When pus has already formed. Stitching pain in the left ovary. General perspiration without relief, chilliness; creeping chilliness; aggravation at night.

Palladium: Swelling and indurations of right ovary. pain in right ovarian region relieved by pressure.

Plus: Ovaritis from suppression of menses after getting feet well; constant chilliness.

Staph: Ovarian affection from masturbation or after prolonged absence of husband.

PARALYSIS

Loss or diminution of the power of voluntary motion in any part of the body. Paralysis means diminution of the power of voluntary motion. Paralysis of one lateral half of the body, usually caused by a lesion in the brain on the opposite side, is called Hemiplegia. When one half of the body taken transversely is paralyzed, the ailment is called Paraplegia, which is generally caused by diseases of the spinal marrow. Shaking palsy goes by the name of Paralysis agitans.

Consult the article on Locomotors ataxia.

Therapeutics Leading Indications

Acon: When caused by exposure to cold, *esp*. dry, cold winds. From violent emotions. Accompanied by a sense of coldness, numbness, and more particularly tingling in the affected part.

Arg-n: Paraplegia after debilitating causes. Staggering gait. Walks and stands unsteadily, *esp*. when he thinks himself unobserved. Debility in Calves.

Bar-c: Paralysis of old people with weakness of memory, great weakness of mind and body: the patient is childish, condition being half imbecile. Palsy of old people. Paralysis following apoplexy, in old people. Who are childish with loss of speech (tongue being paralyzed). *Paralysis of tongue.

Caust: After exposure to dry cold winds, when the affection becomes chronic and after failure of Acon. Which has also paralysis from the same cause, but Acon. is indicated in the beginning. Paralysis of *single part, such as vocal organs, muscles of deglutition, tongue, upper eyelids, face, bladder, extremities; generally right side (Lach. left). Weakness of Caust. Progresses until we have gradually appearing paralysis. Paralysis following typhoid, typhus, diphtheria, rheumatism etc.

Dulc: Paralysis brought on or made worse by cold, damp weather or from sudden changes from hot to cold, after suppression of eruptions or suppression of eruptions from cold (Sulph. may have to be given in alternation). Paralyses of upper and lower limbs. Paralysis of arm which feels icy cold. Paralysis of tongue with impaired speech; involuntary discharge of urine.

Gels: "Complete relaxation or prostration. Or the whole muscular system, with almost or quite entire motor paralysis." Muscles will not obey the will. Hands and the lower extremities rumble on attempting to move; must lie still. Staggering. Partial paralysis of bladder with intermittent flow. Also involuntary urination. Muscles of deglutition paralyzed. Tongue paralyzed: tongue trembles, speech thick. Loss of voice on account of paralysis of laryngeal muscles; can at best whisper.

Lach: Paralysis, generally Left-sided; or semi-lateral (side attacked being immaterial). Both mind and body worn out, with relaxation of muscular face. Following apoplexy. Awkward, stumbling gait. Hot flushes. *Mind worse after sleep.

Merc-s: Paralysis agitans. "Paralysis commence in upper extremities and runs downwards." "Indescribable malaise of the body and soul."

Nux-v: After abuse of alcohol, after sexual excesses, after apoplexy. Incomplete paralysis of arms, legs, with vertigo. feels worse in morning on waking.

Phos: Progressive paralysis as a result of spinal affections. Paralysis after sexual excesses. Paralytic lassitude after a very short walk. Tumbling of limbs from slight exertions.

Plumb: Paralysis of single muscles. Infantile paralysis. Paralysis from over-exertion of extensor muscles, as in piano-players, when, evidently, extension is difficult of impossible, while flexion is sound. Sometimes the flexors are paralyzed. Progressive paralysis. Throat paralyzed; cannot swallow. Paralysis preceded by mental derangement; painful contraction of Limbs with emaciation of the affected parts. Wrist-drop. Obstinate constipation.

Rhus-t: The great anti-paralytic. Particularly useful in rheumatic paralysis with great stiffness, tingling and numbness of affected parts; brought on by exposure to wet, strains or excessive exertion, Paralytic weakness, *esp.* when sitting and at rest. "Lameness in the extremities with stiffness of joints, worse when rising from a seat." "Complete paralysis, hemiplegic or paraplegia, with dragging, slow, difficult gait." Paralytic rigidity in limbs, *remarkably pronounced on first beginning to move. Paralysis of single parts, single limbs. Paralysis of rectum and bladder.

Alumin: One-sided paralysis, *esp.* of the extensors so that he cannot extend the affected limb. "Slow, tottering gait as after severe illness." Unable to walk except with the eyes open and in the daytime; staggers when closing eyes and when walking in the dark. Paralytic weight in arms. Difficulty in swallowing due to paretic condition of esophagus. Paretic condition of bladder. Urine slow to start and slow to flow, and in some cases it dribbles, esophagus feels constricted when swallowing.

Colch: After suddenly checked sweat *esp*. foot-sweat by getting wet. Paralytic pain in arm, cannot hold the slightest thing firmly. "Loss of sensibility of tongue, the first symptom in Colchicum paralysis."

Coni: Palsy of old people *esp*. old women. "Conium may be useful in paralysis, especially partial, the patient being weak and continuously trembling; the limbs continually trembling; the limbs give out when walking and he falls forward; sudden attacks of giddiness and faintness." (cowperth waite). Palsy after concussion of spine.

Stan: Hemiplegic, *esp*. left side, with a feeling of heavy load on arm and corresponding side of the chest; from worms, or onanisn.

PHOTOPHOBIA

Photophobia on intolerance of light is caused by or it associated with some ailment. It should be treated in the light of causation, when causation is known.

Therapeutics Leading Indications

Acon: Excessive photophobia; black spots or mist before eyes.

Arg-n: Photophobia worse in a warm room; suddenly becomes far-sighted.

Arsen: Excessive sensitiveness to light *esp*. to day light.

Bell: With convulsive movements of eyes when light strikes them; light seems to be surrounded by halo divided in various colours.

Lac-d: Even candle-light is unbearable. Dim vision can only see light, not objects.

Silic: Chronic photophobia.

Sulph: Eyes dazzled by day; night-blindness; halo see around a lamp-light.

PHTHISIS (TUBERCULOSIS OF LUNGS)

This is tuberculosis of the lungs. Characterized by: cough of varying severity, finally giving out a toneless sound; constant short hacking cough, later expectoration of glassy, glutinous mucus, sometimes with streaks of yellowish colour which are significant, but what is more characteristic is a tinge or streaks of blood. Profuse expectoration of blood often proves speedily fatal. Other indications are: loss of appetite, diarrhoea, paleness of skin, distinctness of veins, hoarseness or huskiness of voice, pain between the shoulder blades and in the region of the clavicle; moderate fever with copious perspiration; great increase of sexual appetite; brilliant eyes in spite of paleness and emaciation of the other parts of the body. What is very peculiar is that the patient is even to the last sanguine of recovery.

It should be remembered that the good action of a well-selected remedy manifests itself generally by the swelling of glands, rheumatism, hoarseness, pimples and pustules around nose, otorrhoea, headache, toothache, eruptions, piles etc., which should not be disturbed by a change of medicine or repetition.

Therapeutics Leading Indications

Calc-c: One of the greatest remedies in phthisis. Constitutional symptoms of the remedy are guiding in its selection for which refer to Drug-pictures in Silhouette. Called for in a patient who had been during childhood sweaty-headed, pot-bellied, fat, flabby with irregular bone development, sluggish or slow in movement, slow in cutting teeth. Called for in a girl who menstruated too early and too profusely? Tendency to row fat, *esp.* in children or young people; great tendency to take cold; great weakness in ascending, walking, talking. Tendency to diarrhoea, generally worse afternoons. Irregular menstruation, early, too long, too profuse. Painless hoarseness, worse mornings. Sensation of dust or feather in throat, lungs, causing tickling or exciting cough. Shortness of breath and palpitation on going up the slightest ascent. Much rattle of mucus in chest. Fever worse evenings with partial sweat. Pain and rawness in chest while coughing. Fully developed stage: formation of large cavities, *esp.* about middle right lung, pain in middle or right side of chest as if beaten (Arnic); entire chest is painfully sensitive to touch and on inspiration. Rattles of mucus heard over chest, worse right side. Expectoration tough, purulent, yellowish green and bloody; or yellowish, fetid; tastes sweetish; when spat into water falls to the bottom with a "trail of tough mucus behind like a falling star." Great repugnance to animal food.

Ferr-m: Should be given when strongly indicated as otherwise it may aggravate the troubles. Valuable in vomiting of blood in phthisis, *esp.*, in young boys and girls who are in the incipient stage of phthisis Florida. Anaemia, face pale but easily becomes red and flushed on the least pain, emotion or exertion. "Great paleness of mucous membrane, *esp.* that of the cavity of the mouth." (Raue). Nosebleed with bright red flushing of face. Nosebleed alternating with spitting of blood. Profuse menstruation. Pains in chest flying from one point to another. Undigested painless stool at night or while eating or drinking. Relief of symptoms by walking about.

Iodium: In young persons who grow too rapidly, who are subject to frequent congestions to chest and are lean, thin, and dark in complexion; who always feel too hot (it is not febrile heat). Warmth, warm room intolerable. Great weakness, even speaking excites perspiration. Great weakness and loss of breathe ongoing upstairs (Calc-c.). Chronic diarrhoea of an exhaustive character. Eats freely well but loss flesh all the time. Sweats easily and easily becomes exhausted. Dry cough caused by tickling all over chest. Lungs consolidated. (Dr. Behr recommends the 6th potency and adds that the Ist is often indispensable.)

Kali-c: Dyspeptic symptoms (*see* Dyspepsia) precede the development of the disease. the right, *esp.* the lower part of the right lung is affected. Stitching pains may be felt all over chest, at times running right through to back. Expectoration bloody and contains "Pus or globules of pus scattered through it." *Puffiness of upper eyelids. Aggravation of symptoms from three to five a.m. "A very stubborn sensation of chilliness at noon." (Farmington). Kali-c. and Crab-v. complement each other.

Stan: Very sad and feels like crying all the time. Whereas a phthisical patient is hopeful to the least. Hence Farrington says that it is rarely indicated in true tuberculosis. On the basis of my own experience, I venture to place it on record that both Stan. And Bapt. which lack hopefulness so common to phthisical patients, play their role all right even when contra-indicated from the stand-point of a state of despondency. *Great weakness in chest which feels as if it were empty; worse from talking; *so weak, unable to talk, can hardly talk, or talks in a very feeble voice. (This feeble voice is no joke. I had the opportunity of treating a case, in which the patient whispered into my ear what he wanted to express. Stan. Cured the case radically.) While talking, weakness and aching in deltoid and arms. Weakness is felt more when descending stairs than when ascending them. Putrid breath. Excessive weakness of digestion. Excessive emaciation. Very yellow or greenish with a saltish or sweetish taste. Voice deep, hoarse and hollow. Constant chilliness with flushes of heat.

Sulph: Feels constantly too hot; frequent flushes of heat. Alternately cold and burning feet, or cold feet in daytime and burning soles at night. Loss of appetite, drinks much, eats little. Nightly suffocative attacks, wants doors and windows open; becomes suddenly wide awake at night. Diarrhoea during out of bed early in morning. Cough mostly dry, may be loose and rattling. Weakness of chest when talking. "Pain running through left upper chest to scapula." "Pain left side of chest in lower portion through to left shoulder blade."

Tuber. or Bacil: When there is a family history of tuberculosis, Patient is usually sad, despondent, of light complexion narrow chest, emaciated, anemic, tired easily, averse to work. Great weakness in lower extremities, *esp.* form knees down to feet. Loss of appetite *esp.* in morning. *Great emaciation with incredible rapidity. "*Takes cold easily without knowing how and where." *Symptoms change all the time, affecting one organ after another, such as brain, lungs, liver, kidneys, stomach, nervous system etc. Enlarged glands. Pains shift from one place to another, now here and now there, coming and going suddenly. Early morning diarrhoea (Sulph.). Sensation of freezing on back in evening (it may be at any time as I have noticed in a case which was cured with this remedy). *Air hunger. Clothes feel damp. "Not satisfied to remain in one place for a long time; wants to travel." (*N.B.* Hydras. often fattens patient cured with tuber.) *N.B.* Although both the remedies (nosodes) are identical or all practical purposes, Bacil. is called for when there is *excessive mucus purulent bronchial secretion, threatening to occlude the lungs. Both Bacil. and Tuber. are particularly adapted to more chronic cases of Tuberculosis, to the acute stage of which they do not, as a rule, respond.

Acet-ac: *Slow fever with drenching night-sweat. Left cheek very red or red spot of left cheek. Dropsy to feel and legs with intense, insatiable thirst. Great debility. Haemoptisis. Pale Waxen face.

Ars-i: (3X or 6X trit.) Has cured various forms of phthisis in its different stages. Decided cachestic appearance. Hectic fever; tendency to diarrhoea; tightness to chest and difficult expectoration. Expectoration greenish yellow and pus-like.

Calc-p: Incipient phthisis in anemic patients; profuse night sweats; *esp.* about face and neck. Chronic cough with cold extremities. Chronic cough with soreness and dryness of throat. Stitches in chest, *esp.* in right side, with cough. Purulent, greenish expectoration. Swelling of glands. (Tubercular laryngitis.) Involuntary sighing. Weary when going upstairs.

Carb-an: In the late stages: horribly offensive sputum; cold feeling in chest (Brom.). As soon as he closes eyes he feels like smothering. Foul, exhausting night sweats which stain linen yellow.

Carb-v: Particularly in late stages: expectoration very offensive; voice hoarse; weak digestion; great debility from slight exertion; great air hunger; rattling in chest; cold knees in bed at night. Phthisis commences in larynx with painless hoarseness (Calc-c.). Aching pains through apex to right scapula (left, Sulph.).

Caust: In laryngeal phthisis (Dros., Spong., Hepar, Selen.). Great hoarseness, worse morning, with rawness, burning and soreness in chest. See Cough.

Ferr-p: Galloping phthisis. Cough acute, short, spasmodic and very painful. there is blood-streaked expectoration.

Hamam: Haemoptisis; tickling cough with taste blood. Profuse venous blood comes into mouth without coughing or any effort. Unwarranted mental calmness. (I have added the word, unwarranted.) Exhaustion out of all proportionate blood lost, yet the patient exhibits no alarm or anxiety.

Lyco: Adapted to persons who are weak, puny, sickly; intellectually keen but physically weak. Upper part of body emaciated, lower part semidropsical. Ravenous hunger but a small quantity of food fills him right up. Phthisis after badly treated pneumonia: loose cough as if chest were full of mucus with rattling; half-open condition of eyes during sleep; expectoration thick, lemon-yellow; greenish yellow; large quantities of pus; tasting salty; offensive. Hectic fever worse from 4 to 8 p.m. Circumscribed redness of cheeks.

Merc-s: Great aggravation lying on right side in matters relating to cough, vomiting etc., it being often impossible to lie on right side. *See* Cough. *Tongue flabby shows imprint of teeth. *Sticky, profuse sweat without relief. Offensive smell in mouth.

Nat-s: When complicated with old malarial fever Non-tubercular phthisis in sycotic constitutions. Extreme sensitiveness to damp. Feels better in dry weather, hot or cold. Much pains in chest on coughing, *esp.* in lower left lung. Pains about ninth and tenth ribs on left side. Holds chest with hands when coughing, as pressure ameliorates. Painful soreness with loose cough (Bryon., with dry cough).

Puls: It weeps easily; has wandering pains with chilliness; feels oppressed in a warm room, better in open air. Constant internal chilliness even in a warm room. Loss of taste or smell. Dry cough disappearing on sitting up in bed and returning on lying down. Expectoration bitter, yellowish green; streaked with blood; black, clotted blood. When there is a history of serious ailments, such as anaemia, colourists, bronchitis, pneumonia etc. at puberty and she says that she has never been well since. Puls. should be the first medicine to be studied.

Sang: Phthisis Florida. Hemorrhage from lungs during incipient phthisis; *esp*. in women suffering from scanty menstruation; burning and stitches in chest from right side to shoulder; severe oppression of breathing; copious night sweats, which may be cold. Circumscribed redness (hectic flush) of cheeks in afternoon. Breath and sputa smell offensive even to the patient; sputa may be pus-like. Cough at first dry and excited by tickling in larynx and upper part of chest; later loose with profuse expectoration which smells badly even to the patient.

Silic: Slow catarrhal phthisis of old people. In the late stages with expectoration of offensive pus or much-pus when it will have palliative effect, cure being hardly possible. it is called for *esp*. in childhood when the child presents symptoms, which if not checked may tend to development of the disease. This is treating tuberculosis before it is developed to a state recognizable as one of tuberculosis. Here study the constitutional symptoms of Silic., such as, imperfect nourislument, defective assimilation, lack of physical stamina (great weakness of nerves, debility, inclination to lie down, slowness manifested in learning to walk, decided want to vital heat), hungry but cannot eat, offensive foot-sweat, passing of even soft stool with difficulty, chilliness with tendency to catch cold, *esp*. when feet and head are uncovered, body emaciated, while the abdomen is distended. Head disproportionally large, *profuse sour-smelling head-sweat when body is dry etc.

Spong: Phthisis begins in apex of left lung. *See* Cough. Everything seems perfectly dry and light, no mucus with the cough. The patient may be flabby. Weak; feels heavy when walking in open air, must sit down. Feels relieved by lying down quietly. Clears throat constantly. Phthisis of children: Arsen. Expectoration fouls, pus-like.

PLAGUE

An acute infectious and contagious disease. It was unknown in India till 1896 A.D., when it made its way into the country from Hongkong.

Therapeutics Leading Indications

Arsen: Glands of right side predominantly affected. Sudden great weakness with mental restlessness; oppressive shyness of breath.

Anth: May be tried in any case unless some other remedy is indicated. it has rapid loss of strength; fever heart beats frequent but weak, sinking pulse; glands swollen and painful.

Badi: Very useful in plague. Inguinal glands swollen indurates, whole body very sore.

Bapt: Soreness all over; face dark red with besotted expressive indescribable sick feeling all over; air hunger.

Bell: High fever; sweat on covered parts; inflammation and swelling of glands.

Carb-v: Feet and legs icy cold to knees; blueness of skin of lips; sudden prostration.

Lomine: A preparation of the pus of the plague, which has reputation for curing plagues, even when swelling begin to suppurate.

Nit-ac: Sticking or pricking pains in glands; inflammation swelling and suppuration of glands; glands extremely sensitive to touch. All discharge offensive.

Phyto: Glands in armpits enlarged. Glands of right side of neck hard and swollen. Affected glands may feel burning and painful.

Rhus-t: Painful stiffness of glands. It has swelling inguinal glands. Aching all over body. Parotid gland (*esp.* right) swollen, painful, neck being stiff (Stiffness relieved by continued movement of neck.).

Silic: *Esp.* indicated just after suppuration of gland or glands has taken place. In duration and swelling of glands (cervical, parotid, axillaries and inguinal ones) for which also it may be used. Sweats as soon as he falls as sleep.

Sulph-ac: Weakness is inordinate; breath very offensive; lips cracked and exfoliate.

Ver-a: Sudden sinking of strength; extreme prostration; cold sweat on forehead. Fever with external coldness. Craves cool and refreshing thing. Violent inflammation.

PLEURISY

Inflammation of the pleura, the delicate serous membrane which covers the lungs and lines the cavity of the chest. It comes on with chilliness, fever, aching, switching pains in the side which are increased by deep inspiration, coughing and by pressure. May be complicated with bronchitis, pneumonia, measles, tuberculosis etc.

Therapeutics Leading Indications

Acon: Principal remedy which is in most cases sufficient to effect a complete cure. High fever, dry, hot skin, restlessness; violent thirst, red face, shortness of breath. Stitching pains in chest or on a fixed spot of thorax, worse from breathing, coughing, sneezing etc. cannot lie on right side. After mechanical injuries (Arnic.).

Arnic: Feeling as if chest and ribs were bruised. *Sore feeling all over body as from bruises. After mechanical injury.

Bryon: Often called for after Acon. Cough hard painful; phlegm scanty. *Sharp, stitching pains of affected parts, worse from inspiration or slightest motion. Generally, better from lying on affected side (here pressure relieves).

Kali-c: *Violent stitching pains, *esp.* on right side (left side, Arnica., Phos., Squil.). Dry cough worse from 3 to 4 a.m. In tubercular patients. (With Kali-c. the stitching pains are worse from pressure, worse during rest, while Bryon. modalities are opposite to all this.).

Sulph: Sharp stitching pains through left long to back or through chest to left shoulder-blade, worse lying on back. Causes absorption of pleurtic effusion (Apis., Arson.). When the disease does not yield to well-chosen remedy's. When complicated with pneumonia.

Apis: Well-marked pleurisy effusion refusing to be absorbed, with oppression and fiendishness, feeling as if he would be unable to breathe again. Cough worse in warn room; face oedematous; scanty urine; moderate fever.

Arsen: Profuse serous effusion. Protracted case with extreme prostration, great oppression of breathing rapid respiration, worse on attempting of lie down.

Merc-s: Violent fever, frequent chills, *esp.* creeping chilliness followed by burning heat; sweats without relieved impossible to lie of right side; cough increased by lying right side.

Nit-ac: Pleurisy of old people or in broken-down constitutions. Chilly. Pricking (splinter-like) pains affected parts; pains excited by touch and lightest jar. Snatches in right side of chest.

Seneg: *Esp.* indicated in fat persons. When there is burning in chest, either before or after coughing. Difficult breathing with sensation as if chest were too tight and burning in chest.

Squilla: Difficult breathing with stitching pains on left side; worse during inspiration. Stitches in chest *esp.* when inhaling or coughing. Oppression and tightness in chest. Inability to lie on left side.

PNEUMONIA

Inflammation of lungs, a dangerous malady, no doubt, but easily amenable to homoeopathic treatment. The action of indicated remedies is something more marvelous than one can imagine, be he a layman or a physician. What should be known by the people at large is that a cure under homoeopathy is radical and leaves no chance for recurrence of the disease in a patient homeopathically treated.

Usually sets in with a chill, followed by fever and cough which is at first dry. Later on, tough and tenacious mucus is expectorated with some difficulty. Frequently the colour of sputum is like that of iron rust. There is deep-seated dull pain in chest with difficulty breathing.

Stethoscope reveals in the first stage fine crepitation which has been compared to the sound produced by the rubbing of a lock of hair close to the ear.

Therapeutics Leading Indications

Ant-t: *Great rattling and chest full of mucus, as if much would be expectorated but nothing comes up. If expectoration takes place at all, it affords great relief. Suffocative shortness of breath. Cold clammy sweat with great faintness. Consciousness wanes on closing eyes. Thirstlesness or may drink little and often. Nostrils dilate and contract or there may be widely dilated nostrils. Edges of eyelids covered with mucus. Face pale, cyanotic. In some cases prostration may be so great what the patient is noticed slipping down in bed. Pneumonia of right lunge, associated with jaundice.

Bryon: Frequently indicated after such remedies as Acon., Bell., Ferrr-p. etc. have abated fever and perhaps pain to a certain extent in the first stage. Patient wants to lie on affected (painful) side (rev. of Bell.). Cracked or parched; tongue dry. Cough hard and painful, hurts distant parts of body. Stitching pain in chest. Sputa yellow or of soft-brick shade. (very often Sulph. is called for after Bryon. to complete absorption and cure.).

Carb-v: In third stage. Great prostration; patient cyanotic; skin cold, cold knees even in bed; great difficulty in breathing: *wants to be fanned all the time. Pulse thread-like, hardly perceptible, and intermittent. Eyes half-open; hardly perceptible, and intermittent. Eyes half-open; conscious or unconscious. Breathe of foul smell. Abdomen distended with gas.

Chel: Bilious pneumonia, yellow face and skin jaundiced, pain in liver and under right shoulder blade. Stitches in chest, worse right side. Short and oppressed breathing. *Fan-like motion of wings of nose (Lyco., Phos.). One foot cold, the other hot (Lyco.).

Phos: *Esp.* with typhoid symptoms. Great oppression and tightness of chest. Dry cough and rust-coloured sputa, of bloody mucus. Cough hurts and makes him tremble, worse lying on left side. "Moans and grunts with every breath and suppresses cough by it, just as he can, because it hurts him so." Lying on left side aggravates symptoms. Burning thirst for ice-cold water. *Esp.* called for when lower lobe of right lung is affected.

Rhus-t: With typhoid symptoms. Low mild delirium with stupefaction. Excessive restlessness with tossing about. *Dry tongue with triangular red rip. Lying still aggravates pain and oppression of breathing. Sputa of brick dust colour or bloody.

Arsen: In advanced stages. Great anxiety with tossing about. Great fear of death. Face pale, cold extremities, great prostration. Worse at night, *esp.* after midnight.

Bell: Pneumonia presenting typhoid symptoms in the beginning. Drowsiness with delirium; starts from sleep. Eyes red; face dark red and bloated; upper lips bloated. Fever with sweats on covered parts.

Brom: Lower lobe of right lung affected. Sensation as if he could not get sufficient air into chest. Stitches in right side of chest. Nosebleed.

Carb-a: Late stages of the disease. Expectoration green, purulent and horribly offensive; coming generally from right lung. Oppressed breathing. Sensation of cold in chest.

Ferr-p: In first stage, also in the beginning of the second stage (That of exudation). High fever with moderate anxiety and restlessness. Chest feels sore and bruised. Expectoration scanty and streaked with blood or profuse expectoration of almost pure blood.

Hepar: When pus forms. Pricking pain in chest. Rattling of mucus in chest. Sweats easily.

Kali-c: Stitching pains in chest, *esp.* running through lower part of right chest to hack; wheezing and rattling breathing; great accumulation of mucus in chest, but difficult to expectorate; intense oppression of breathing. *N.B.* Stitching pains of Kali-c. May occur or become aggravated whether the patient moves or not (bryos. stitches worse from motion); with Kali-c: stitching pains and worse during rest and lying on affected side (that is, worse from pressure), Bryon. stitching pains being relieved by pressure. Lastly, Kali-c. stitching pains may occur all over chest, but they occur characteristically in the lower portion of right chest.

Kali-iod: Sputa frothy like soap-suds or profuse, purulent and green. When hepatization has commenced. Great difficulty of berthing.

Lach: In late stage of pneumonia when it assumes a typhoid form, *esp.* when abscess forms in lungs. Low muttering delirium. sputum frothy, purulent, mixed with blood. Hepatization mostly of left lung. Great difficulty of breathing, worse after sleep. Sensation of constriction in chest.

Merc-s: With bilious symptoms, jaundice, great tenderness in region of liver. Oppressed breathing with stitches in right chest. Sputum may be bloody streaked. Worse from lying on right side. Profuse sweat without relief. Flabby tongue taking imprint of teeth. Most uncomfortable from warmth of bed.

Opium: Pneumonia of old topers. *Deep snoring breathing with wide-open mouth. Hot sweat all over body (excepting lower limbs). Coldness of extremities. Bed feels too hot. "He gropes with his hands about the bed as though he were hunting something." (Bernreuter).

Sang: Second and third stage. Typhoid pneumonia. Second stage: tough and rust-coloured sputa, difficult to rise. Third stage: sputa pus-lie and offensive, selling very badly even to the patient. Sharp stitching pains, *esp.* about right lung. Difficulty of breathing very distressing. Lies upon his back with head well-elevated. Circumscribed redness of cheeks, *esp.* in afternoon.

POLYPUS

Fleshy or fibrous excrescences very often form in nose, *esp.* in the children.

Therapeutics Leading Indications

Teuc: An all round remedy for Polypus. *Polypus in nose. Polypus with stoppage of nose on side lain on. "Sensation as if the nostrils were stopped; blowing nose or sneezing does not remove obstruction (strict.)." Polypus in uterus or vagina. Fibrous tumors of eyelids, *esp.* inside lower lid. Excrescences in urethra following gonorrhea (removed by injections of the mother tincture of the remedy). Teue. Polypus at times occupy entire right nostril projecting slightly. Teuc for nasal polypus are: Calc-c., Phos., Sang., Silic, Phos. Polypus in nose is apt to bleed easily and with Phos. there is frequent sneezing, foul imaginary smells in nose and also fetid exhalation from nose.

Sang: Polypus on mucous surfaces. Mucus polypus which tends to bleed, Nasal polypus may be associated with alternately fluent and dry coryza or acrid coryza.

Silic: May be tried when other remedies have failed in nasal polypus. it has inflammation in nostrils.

Calc-c: Polypus in nose associated with loss of smell.

Calc-p: Large, pedunculated polypus.

For polypus in ears we have: 1. Calc-c., Lach., Hydras., Teuc., Thuja. 2. Kali-s., Lyco., Phos., Merc-s. Calc-c. has polypus in ears which may be associated with humming and buzzing in ears and sensation, at intervals, of stoppage in ears and hardness of hearing. Lach. has polypus in left ears which may be sensitive to wind. Hydras. has exuberant polypoid growths in ears. Thuja has polypus in middle ear (chronic othitis media). Teuc. is *esp.* adapted to old and middle aged women. Kali-s. Has polypoid excrescence closing meatus near opening of right ear. Merc-c. has polypus in external meatus which is inflamed.

For polypus in uterus, the most prominent remedies are: Calc-c., Calc-p., Coni., Phos., Teuc., Thjua. Teuc. has already been dealt with. Thuja is likely to cure many cases. Conium polypus of uterus protrudes during stool. Polypus in rectum: Many cases yield to Calc-p. Others by Nit-ac., and Phos. The polypi of these two remedies may bleed.

Polypus in larynx: Sang., Thuja.

POST-PARTUM HAEMORRHAGE

By this is meant hemorrhage after delivery.

Therapeutics Leading Indications

Arnic: A few doses of Arnica. 30 administered after delivery are powerful enough to prevent such hemorrhage. It is also called for in such hemorrhage, *esp.* when the whole body feels sore. Also when there is sensation of agitation and trembling of the body. Great prostration.

Bell: Blood feels hot as it passes through vagina. Hourglass contraction. Refer to Placenta, retention of.

Caul: Retained placenta from weakness and exhaustion; flooding from inertia of uterus.

Hyos: Bright blood; more blood is discharge with every start. Flow bright red and steady.

Cinnamonum: Repeated small haemorrhage during gestation and puerperal state; worse from exertion. Haemorrhage of this remedy takes place some days after delivery.

Croc: Post-partum haemorrhages. Black and slimy blood. Bleeding in large clots. Bleeding excited by the least movement.

Nux-m: Hemorrhage continued and obstinate. Flow thick and dark. Pressure in abdomen.

Sabin: Flow painless, of dark red blood. Flow takes place in gushes; abates only to reappear in outburst. Pains extend from sacrum to pubes.

Thlaspi: Profuse flow, blood dark red and clotted; violent uterine colic and cramps.

PUERPERAL FEVER

Therapeutics Leading Indications

Bapt: Of septic origin with typhoid symptoms. *see* Typhoid fever.

Bell: Great tenderness of abdomen after delivery; *sensitiveness to slightest jar. Pains in abdomen come on suddenly and disappear suddenly. Flushed face, sweat on covered.

Kreos: Very offensive, excoriating lochia; distension of abdomen; yawning. Patient feels better from warmth.

Rhus-t: Lochia thin and offensive. Inflammation of uterus after confinement; typhoid symptoms. (*see* Typhoid Fever and also Fever, Simple.).

Carb-ac: Remittent fever in autumn. Dusky *face. *Horribly offensive breath; offensive odour from skin. Stool thin, very offensive. Constant yawning. Cold odour hands and feet. Great flatulent distension of abdomen, belching of wind and desire for stimulants.

Crotal: Dangerous malignant type of remittent fever. Often based on a previous low state of the system. Yellow colour of eyes. Fetid breath; cold extremities; symptoms worse after sleep. Diarrhoea; stool black, thin or like coffee-grounds; offensive.

Eup-perf: Remittent fever, *esp*. if occurring in summer and autumn, attended by severe bilious symptoms. See Influenza and Intermittent Fever. Insatiable thirst, but drinking excites nausea and vomiting; vomiting of bitter fluid and bile; aggravated by drinking. Great weakness during fever. Stretching and yawning.

Gels: Dull, drowsy, prostrated, desirous of lying still, of being left alone, apathetic regarding his illness. Aching, sore, bruised feeling in body. Little or no thirst. Constant yawning. Feels heavy and tired.

Merc-s: Alternate chill and heat. Flabby tongue, taking imprint of teeth. Great thirst with moist mouth. Hurried and rapid speech.

Rhus-t: *See* Fever, Simple. White coating only on one side of tongue. Coldness but does not mind cold air. Brain feels loose when shaking head. Craves cold water. But is vomited immediately.

Infantile remittent fever: Acon., Bell., Bryon., Cham., Ipec., Mur-ac., Podo., Puls, Rhust-t.

RENAL COLIC

An urinary stone usually originates in the kidney and there from passes down the ureter into the bladder, causing excruciating pain during its passage along the ureter, ceasing as it reaches the bladder. The violent pain is known as renal colic. Sometimes, however, when a stone attains a size too large for its passage along the ureter, it remains in the kidney causing more or less pain, or no pain at all for years. Hereditary gout or rheumatism plays an important role in the formation of these concretions.

Therapeutics Leading Indications

Berb: Sticking, digging, tearing or pulsative pains in region of one kidney or both, worse from deep pressure, extending from kidney to bladder and urethra, with urging to urinate. Renal colic worse left side. Urination accompanied by pains in thighs and loins. Backache with severe prostration.

Calc-c: Is said to have power to expel renal stone and also stone in bladder. urine red like blood or brownish red with white and mealy sediment. Urine after standing looks like lime-water; burning in urethra during urination.

Calc-renalis: One of the important medicines having reputation for expelling renal calculi or vesicle calculi (that is, stone in bladder). Lower trifurcation to be taken for a long time it is desired to put a stop to the formation of such stones.

Lyco: A great remedy to correct the disposition to urinary calculi and for expelling renal calculi or renal gravels (of the size of the pinhead, calculi bring or larger size). Severe backache relieved by passing urine. See kidney affections.

Sars: Urine charged with gravel or small pebbles. "Where the patient has gravel and there is considerable deposit in the urine which looks like grey sand; also pus in the urine." Blood in urine towards the conculsion of urination. Great pain is experienced near the neck of bladder, *soon after an emission of urine (that is, just at the end of urination). Child screams before and during urination, sand in urine or on diaper.

Arnic: Agonizing pain in back and hips from passage of calculi. Brick-dust sediment in urine.

Benz-ac: With gout. Kidney pain penetrated chest. Dark brown sediment in urine.

China: Urine with brick red sediment. Contains crystals of urates, oxalates etc.

Nit-ac: Urinary calculi consisting of calcium oxalate. Red sand or sediment in urine. Urine is cold when it is passed. Urine scanty, dark-brown; smelling intolerably, strong like horse's; or extremely offensive.

Pariera: Urine contains much viscid, thick, whitish mucus, or deposit of red sand; smells strongly of ammonia.

Sepia: Turbid urine with red, sandy, or brick-coloured sediment. (Urine very offensive.)

Silic: Reddish sand or yellow, gritty sediment in urine. Strangury.

Uva-ursi: Calculi in bladder, flow of urine stops suddenly as if a stone has rolled suddenly in front of internal orifice or urethra. Urine ropy and bloody. Painful suddenly in front of internal orifice or urethra. Urine copy and bloody. Painful urination with burning sensation. Burning and tearing pains in region of bladder.

RHEUMATISM

Therapeutics Leading Indications

Act-r: In muscles of back and neck; feeling of stiffness and contraction. Head drawn back from contraction of muscles at the nape. Violent aching drawn back. Articular rheumatism of the lower extremities with much swelling and heat of affected parts; pain worse from motion extorting cries. *Esp.* indicated in nervous hysterical women suffering from uterine diseases.

Bryon: *Esp.* useful in muscular rheumatism, muscles inflamed, sore to touch, painful, sometimes swollen, worse from motion. Rheumatism of joints; pain and swelling do not change locality at all or change very slowly. *Esp.* of large joints; violent local inflammation; affected parts swollen, hot, shining red, dark or pale red; better from warmth; worse from motion, also from constipation.

Colch: Rheumatism shifting from one joint to another. Such shifting pains may be wave-like. Pains go from left to right. Or begins in one side of body and flies to the other. Worse in damp, cold weather; great sensitiveness to touch; worse from motion. Now add: without swelling or with moderate swelling; parts dark or pale red; urine dark pale and scanty; constant chilliness even near oven. Remember: Colch. pains are extremely acute and unbearable.

Ledum: Smaller joints mostly affected. Rheumatic pains in lower extremities, *esp.*, in hip and knee-joints, pains commencing in lower limbs and travelling upwards. Pains shoot upwards. Rheumatic inflammation of great. Toe; hot swelling of hip and shoulder joints. Pains worse from motion, at night, from warmth of bed and bed covering. *Better from cold application or only when holding feet in ice-water. From abuse of alcohol.

Puls: *Pains shift (rapidly) from one part to another or attack only one side. Rheumatism of joints; of small of back which feels as if dislocated; of gonorrheal origin.

Arnic: Parts feel sore and bruised; fears even the possibility of being struck by persons coming near.

Bell: Red, shunning, swelling of joints; tearing cutting pain deep in bone; worse from touch and slightest motion and a night; high fever. Pains come on suddenly and disappear suddenly.

Caul: Erratic pains (which change place every few minutes). Pains shift from extremities to back and nape of neck, with rigidity of muscles where they end (neck of back). Rheumatism of women, *esp.* of small joints, such as fingers, wrists, toes, ankles etc. with considerable swelling, erratic pains and painful stiffness of affected joints. Joints crack when walking or turning. Rheumatism in conjunction with uterine or ovarian troubles. Rheumatism alternating with asthma.

Caust: With contraction and stiffness of joints; tension and shortening of muscles. Must move constantly but motion do not relieve. "Chronic articular rheumatism, when joints are stiff and tendons are shortened, drawing the limbs out of shape, worse from cold and better from warmth." (Guaiacum has all these symptoms, but it has aggravations from attempt at motion.)

Dulc: After exposure to wet weather or weather suddenly changing to damp cold, or aggravation from every cold change of the weather. Rheumatism from suppressed sweet or skin diseases.

Ferr-m: Rheumatism of left shoulder and deltoid. Pains relieved by slowly moving about.

Guaiac: Drawing, tension and contraction in tendons, drawing limbs out of shape (some similarity with Caust. after which it follows well). Warmth and motion aggravate pain in joints, cold relieves it. Rheumatic pains in upper arm and shoulder. Rheumatic stiffness of back of neck and back.

Lac-c: Wandering rheumatic pains, which constantly fly from one part to another. Rheumatism alternates sides every few hours or days. For instance, it may attack one ankle first and then the other, and then comes back again to the original locality; in this way it may attack knees, hips and shoulders.

Lyco: Chronic rheumatism, *esp*. of old people, worse at rest and damp weather; better from slow motion and warmth; right side principally affected. Urine contains sediment of red sand.

Merc-s: Tearing pains worse at night, from warmth of bed. *Much sweating affording no relief. Puffy swelling, pale or slightly pinkish.

Phyt: Rheumatism of heels with soreness of (left) shoulder (*esp*. in syphilitics). Pains fly from one place to another like electric shocks. Periosteal rheumatism. With syphilitic taint. Pains in middle of long bones. Worse at night and in damp weather.

Rhod: Rheumatic pains which are excited or aggravated by cold, damp, windy weather. Pains worse during rest; during rest pains may be most violent. Pains and stiffness relieved on commencing to move, by continued motion. Relief from warm wrapping. Chronic rheumatism affecting the smaller joints and their ligaments. Rheumatism of knee joint; acts best of right side is affected.

Silic: Chronic hereditary rheumatism; pains worse at night and from uncovering (Ledum, reverse); better from warmth. Constitutional symptoms are guiding.

Thuja: Of syphilitic or gonorrheal origin. Articular rheumatism following suppression of gonorrheal discharge. Sweating of uncovered parts. Coldness and numbness of affected parts. pain worse in warm room. Left side, *esp*. affected. The patient is chilly and sensitive to cold, damp air.

RINGWORM

Characterized by itchy pimples operating in circular form. Ringworms of the scalp, body and beard are respectively known as Tinea sodium, Herpes Circinnatus and Sycosis.

Therapeutics Leading Indications

Bar-c: "Ringworm in children subject to glandular swellings on various parts of the body, face excepted." Excoriation and oozing. (Excoriation and oozing between scrotum and thighs.)

Clem: Insupportable itching from warmth of bed and after washing. Eruptions moist while the *moon is increasing. and pale and dry when the moon is waning.

Nat-m: Often useful in herpes Cincinnatus (Sepia, Bar-c., Tell.) Face of the patient pale, shining, greasy looking. Psoric tuberculosis patient. Symptoms worse in heat of summer. Feels better in open air. There is a great desire for open and for washing in cold water.

Phyt: With syphilitic taint. With chronic gonorrheal affections. Worse from the warmth of bed; itching worse forepart of night, preventing sleep till midnight. Worse in damp weather and washing.

Sepia: Ringworm in isolated spots on upper part of body. Ringworm-like eruptions every spring on different parts of body. Dry ringworm on face. Relief from warmth of bed or hot applications. Itching not relieved by scratching and it apt to change to burning.

Tell: A great remedy for ringworm. Ringworm *esp.* of the face and body (often over a great portion of body or whole body). More pronounced on lower limbs. Body thickly covered with elevated rings or ringworms, *esp.* on legs. Rings intersecting at places in a crowded way, thereby making its specific character. Ringworm on scrotum and perineum. (*N.B.* I feel disinclined to lay any particular stress on the words "lower limbs" and "*esp.* on legs", as previously noted. From the number of cases treated by me with Tellurium alone, I am led to conclude that the remedy is sharply indicated in cases where the whole of the upper part of the body (face may not be affected at all) is covered with ringworm in crowded manner. Now then, let me add; "Ringworm at any part of the body, red, elevated rings very distinctly marked with minute itching vesicles *esp.* on lower extremities, worse at night, after going to bed; vesicles filled with a watery excoriating fluid smelling like fish-brine."—Bhanja.

Arsen: Ringworm on scalp: dry and rough hair falling out in patches.

Chrysophanic acid: Particularly, 3X trit. for internal administration and also ointment prepared with Vaseline for external use has been found to cure ringworms. The 3X trit. Given internally alone produced wonderful effect in a few cases under my treatment. I never prescribed it for external application.

Dulc: With fetid sweat.

Nat-c. Herpes circinatus: skin dry, rough and chapped; dryness of skin with profuse sweat from least exercise or slightest labour.

SALIVATION

Therapeutics Leading Indications

Amm-c: Accumulation of much saliva in mouth and constant spitting.

Arum-t: Excessive salivation; acrid saliva.

Bryon: Accumulation of soapy and frothy saliva in mouth Putrid smell of mouth.

Cham: Frothy saliva; putrid smell of mouth.

Dulc: Accumulation of Silva. Saliva may by tenacious or soap-like. Rheumatic salivation, caused by sleeping under as open window.

Graph: Excessive accumulation of saliva in the Moring. Accumulation of mucus in palate and throat.

Hepar: Accumulation of water in mouth. Patient extremely sensitive to cold air.

Ipec: Profuse salivation. Constantly bilged to swallow saliva. Salivation with lying.

Iris: Profuse flow of Saliva; water drops from mouth when talking.

Kali-i: Copious salivation with nausea. Bloody saliva with disgusting taste.

Lyco: Accumulation of water in mouth; putrid odour from mouth, *esp.* in morning on waking; hungry but speedy satiety.

Nit-ac: Profuse flow of saliva which has fouled odour. Saliva bloody in morning.

Nux-v: Nocturnal salivation. Saliva is bloody. Dryness of mouth but with much accumulation of saliva in fauces. Bad taste in mouth in morning. Salivation with qualmishness.

Puls: Accumulation of sweet saliva in the mouth. watery saliva, like water brash. Sometimes there is inclination to vomit. Or constant spitting of frothy, Cotton-like mucus. Bad taste in mouth in morning.

Sepia: Saline salivation. Fetid breath; Fetid urine, Dryness of mouth. Lips and tongue.

SCABIES

Contagious eruptions on the skin caused by parasites called "aearus" which burrow themselves into the skin, where they lay their eggs and multiply causing inflammation and producing pustules, and vesicles filled with a serous fluid. They appear most frequently about the wrists and between the fingers.

In the opinion of many homoeopaths, true acarus itch is not a constitutional disease as no constitutional disturbance results from curing itches by external applications. Dr. Baehr says: "We hold that all treatment of the itch, as long as the acarus is not extirpated, is downright absurdity." Dr. Farrington says; "You are justified in using as a local application anything that will kill the insect, but not suppress the disease. Such an application you have in Oil of Lavender, which kills both the insects and their ova."

To me it seems that truth lies somewhere in the middle and that the same principles do not hold good in combating all cases of scabies. Let me simply state that while local application of some efficacious ointment is curative in certain cases, it is absolutely useless in tackling the malady in others.

Space at my disposal forbids me to enter into details. Let me, therefore, simply state one case only.

A gentleman has been suffering from most exasperating type of itches all over fingers, wrists and thighs. He has recourse to all sorts of ointments without deriving any good result there from. At long last, after undergoing the trouble for nearly a month, he had one day high sympathetic fever and the eruptions looked rather ferocious, if I may say so; swelling, inflammation, exudation, and pain (burning) rose to a climax. At this stage I was called to give immediate relief to the patient and then cure the disease radically. I prescribed three doses of Anthracinum 30 which were to be taken every half an hour. The effect was both astonishingly speedy and decisive. After 24 hours the itches lost all their virulence. After waiting for full one day, Croton-1. 30 and then the same medicine in the 200th potency were prescribed. Within 5 to 6 days, the disease left no trace behind. These two remedies are rather conspicuous by their absence in our therapeutics.

SCIATICA

Neuralgia affecting the sciatic nerves running from the nates to the ankles. The entire length of the nerve may or may not be affected. The pain is due to tension of the sciatic nerve.

Therapeutics Leading Indications

Amm-m: Pain in left hip as if tendons were too short; limps while walking due to this tension; gnawing pain in bones while sitting. Pains worse while sitting, slightly relieved while walking and entirely relieved while lying down.

Bell: Pain in hip-joint *esp.* at night; has to change position often. Worse from least jar. Better from letting the limb hang down, warmth and in an erect posture.

Cham: *Esp*. left side affected; violent drawing, tearing pains, *numb feeling pain in affected parts; pain worse at night in bed and from motion.

Coloc: Tearing pains shoot down from hip to thigh, leg and feet; crimpy pains in hip of if screwed in a vise, lies upon affected side with knees drawn up; shooting pain like lightning down the whole limbs; sciatica. *Esp*. of right side (may be of left): pains set in suddenly, are constant in character, becomes intolerable in paroxysms. Worse from touch, cold, motion; better during perfect rest, and from pressure, warmth. Note that pressure gives relief at first, but later on pressure aggravates pain.

Eup-perf: Severe shooting pains in course of left sciatic nerve, producing a palsied sensation, *esp*. after motion; gnawing in hip-bone; legs feels tired, particularly left.

Hyper: Sciatica; from injury to nerve. Excruciating pain. Worse from damp weather.

Ignat: when associated with chilliness; of intermittent character; occurring every day or every other day; better in summer, worse in winter. Chronic (Lyco., Sulph.).

Mag-p: Paroxysms violent, lighting-like shocks, worse right side; pains extort cries. Worse from touch, cold air, pressure; better from external heat.

Ledum: Pain begins in foot and runs upwards. Affected limbs cooler than rest of body. Pains worse in bed when getting warm. Great tenderness of soles of feet. General coldness and chilliness.

Phyt: neuralgic pain on outer side of thigh; desire to move but any attempt at moving aggravates pain. Pains fly like electric shocks; of a shooting character; appear and disappear suddenly, Syphilitic taint.

Rhus-t: When caused by exposure to wet or straining in lifting. Pain is attended with numbness, formication and paralytic stiffness of the affected limb; worse during rest and when beginning to move; relieved for a short time by motion; relief from heat and rubbing.

Ruta: Deep-seated in as if in marrow of bone; worse at rest; pain compell patient to walk about constantly during paroxysm. After injuries, contusions etc.

Still: Left-sided seiatica, of syphilitic origin. Sciatica of gonorrheal orig. Pain may be much aggravated by exposing parts to cold or even to air. This aggravated condition may be relieved only by covering with flannel or by getting into bed (that is by covering of bed-clothes).

Arnic: From over-exertion, lifting, straining (Rhus-t.). Changes position constantly, as everything on which he lies seems too hard.

Calc-c: From working in water. Pains start from small of back, extend down lower limbs and deep them in constant uneasiness. Stiffness and contraction of limbs. Cramp like pains. Worse at new moon; at full moon.

Caust: Tendons of knees feel too short; feel stiff and contracted; constant desire to move the foot, but motion does not relieve. *Esp.* effects right side. Worse in open air; better from warmth; from warmth of bed.

Dios: Pain is right leg from point of exit of sciatic nerve, felt only when moving the limb or when sitting up (rising from lying to sitting posture). That means: aggravated by walking or moving the limb and entire relief when sitting still. A few distinct pointers (as I think):

(1) Pains radiate downwards. (2) Frequent shooting pains from one part to another. (3) Pains of all sorts which are unbearable. (4) Pains dart about (go away suddenly and reappear in a different part of the affected limb). *N.B.* Dios. Sciatica may be relieved by stretching the limb and by moving about (he is compelled to walk even though tired, as he cannot afford to sit still).

Ferr-m: Pains relieved while walking slowly about (although weakness, if produced by the disease, obliges the patient to lie down). Pain worse at night, driving or of bed; can hardly put his foot on the ground, but while slowly walking about, pain gradually becomes milder.

Gnaph: Numbness alternating with pain; intense darting. Burning pain along posterior sciatic nerve; worse lying down; worse from motion; better sitting in chair; right side is more affected. Pains may extend to toes.

Hepar: Pain worse from motion, touch and exposure to air: better from being warped up, rest and heat.

Kali-bi: Of left leg, better from walking and flexing leg; worse standing, sitting or lying in bed.

Lach: Pain constantly changes locality, now in head, now in teeth, now in sciatic nerve, attended with nervousness and palpitation of heart.

Merc-s: Tearing pain in hip-joint and knee, worse at night: Chilliness; sweat affording no relief; syphilitic taint.

Nat-m: wrenching pain in hip with shooting. Drawing pains in thighs, knees and legs. Painful contraction of hamstrings. Originating in intermittent fever and abuse of quinine.

Nux-v: Drawing tearing pains from below upwards (Ledum) relief from hot application; can lie best on painless side (reverse of Bryon.); worse early in morning.

Puls: A case declared as hopeless was completely cured by me with Puls. 30 and 200 alone. He was wrongly given Rhus-t. the sharp symptoms were: Left-sided sciatica. Pains worse on beginning to move; relieved by gentle motion (that is, by slowly walking about); better by rubbing and from pressure. Now add: worse evening, night; worse in warm room; worse letting the affected limb hang down; better in open air.

SEA-SICKNESS, RAIN-SICKNESS

Characterized by great nausea, vomiting and vertigo. The best preventive remedies before undertaking voyage or journey by car train are: Coccul., Nux-v., and Petrol. During sickness, the remedies that are remarkably helpful are: Coccul., Nux., Opium, Patrol., Tabac. Dr. Herring says that Opium has afforded quickest relief.

Therapeutics Leading Indications

Coccul: Nausea and vomiting *from riding in carriage, boat, on board ship. Giddiness as if intoxicated.

Nux-v: Disordered stomach either before or during voyage.

Opium: Hot, sweltering sweat or cold sweat on forehead. Voice becomes low and weak. Relaxation of muscles.

Petrol: Face pale and dizziness even in bed. Hering recommends this remedy when Coccul. fails.

Tabac: Sea-sickness: *better on deck, in fresh cold air; with deathly nausea, pallor, coldness; body may be covered with cold sweat. Remember: Deathly nausea, giddiness, vomiting (which may be violent * with cold sweat); dreadful faint feeling of stomach.

Arnic: Sudden onset of the disorder; general prostration of strength. Persons who are easily made train-sick or sea-sick should better take a dose or two of Arnic 30 or 200, one or two days before undertaking travel at an interval of 24 hours.

SMALLPOX

A highly contagious and infectious disease, the period of incubation being about 21 days. Begins with high fever, headache, a bruised pain all over body nut particularly in the small of back. Characteristic Vesicular eruptions are depressed in the centre (a chicken-pox vesicle being pointed in the centre). On about the 8th or 9th day, these vesicles change to pustules containing yellowish matter. These pustules, so long as they are not fully ripe, are also depressed in the centre. These pustules are surrounded by a rose red areola. Vesicles of chicken pox seldom change to pustules and, when so changed, are never surrounded by a red areola.

Now, fever which abated considerably after the full development of eruptions, break out again. The period from the eight to the eleventh day is the most critical one. On the tenth day areola begins to fade. The pustules now generally burst and then crusts are formed which finally fall off in the course of four or five days.

After everything has faded away what remains is called 'pit', being the permanent mark.

The complications of small-pox are numerous. These may be bronchitis, pneumonia, pleurisies, glandular and dropsical swellings, swelling of eyelids etc.

Homoeopathic Prophylactics

Variolinum: "As a preventive of or protection. Against small-pox, it is far superior to crude vaccination and absolutely safe from the sequelae, especially septic and tubercular infection." (Allen)

Vaccininum: A dose of the 6X trit. of the remedy is a "Homoeopathic vaccination having, it is claimed by competent observers, for more prophylactic power against small-pox than vaccination, and none of its dangers or disagreobleness."

Malan: In my opinion the best protective remedy against small-pox. I have verified this hundreds of times. In many cases I had the opportunity to observe that after the administration of a single dose of Maland 30, a few days before vaccination, it did not 'take'. During an epidemic, two or three doses of Maland 30 may profitably be administered at an interval of a week in each case. That is quite sufficient to ward off infection. It is also called for in combating ill-effects of vaccination (Thuja). Skin getting dry and harsh after vaccination calls for Maland.

Treatment of Small-pox

Ant-t: At the commencement when there is great pain in small of back. There may also be yawning and stretching of limbs. (Author). Dry, teasing cough before appearance of eruptions indicates the remedy (Farrington), Ant-t. has pustule eruption closely resembling those of small-pox and, therefore, it is expected to cure them, *esp.* when there is great drowsiness, suffocative shortness of breath. When eruptions partially come out or have been repelled and other symptoms are: great drowsiness; difficulty of breathing; much rattling of mucus in chest but little or nothing comes out.

Bell: During first stage with high fever, flushed face, throbbing headache, sore throat, sweat on covered parts, Pain in back as if it would break or as if dislocated.

Malandrinum: "Prevents or lessens the secondary fever and takes away all offensive exhalation." (Raue). It is apt to play its role in almost all stages of the disease. Nevertheless a few symptoms are: pain along back, as if beaten; cadaverous-smelling stool; dizziness.

Merc-s: *Esp*. during maturation stage, with general symptoms of the remedy.

Hydras: A useful remedy in all stages of small-pox (to use internally as well as externally). Itching and tingling of eruptions; faintness and great prostration. Intense aching in small of back, legs weak and ache. Is said to prevent pitting to a great degree (Act-r., Thuja).

Thuja: Useful in eruptive as well as suppurative stage. I have found it drying up eruptions within two or three days. Two doses of Thuja 30 were given per day for two days only. At all events, it shorten; the course of the disease and prevents pitting.

SNUFFLES

Stoppage of nose with or without coryza. Children are generally affected with this trouble.

Therapeutics Leading Indications

Amm-c: *Stoppage of nose mostly at night; must breathe through mouth (Nux-v.). Without any cold. Starts up every time the child tries to go to sleep.

Nux-v: Coryza fluent during day; stopped at night; nose dry and stuffed; breathes through mouth. "Coryza prevents infants from breathing while nursing; worse at night and towards morning."

Samb: "Child suddenly awakens nearly suffocated, sits up in bed and turns blue; grapes for breath, which it finally gets, then lies down again in bed, to be aroused again sooner or later by another spell." "Nose perfectly dry and completely obstructed. Preventing breathing and nursing; (Chlorine, Mephitis). Oedematous swelling in nose giving rise to snuffles.

Sticta: Nose stuffed up. Constant need or inclination to blow nose, but nothing is discharged; excessive dryness of nose. (Tertiary syphilis.)

Cham: Nose runs, yet stuffed; one cheek red, the other pale; characteristic irritability.

SORE NIPPLES

Arnic: Nipple feel sore and bruised.

Chem: "Nipples inflamed and tender; can hardly endure the pain of nursing; milk cheesy, thickened, mixed with pus."

Graph: Painful and sore nipples with ulcers oozing a thick glutinous fluid; cracks on nipples.

Merc-s: Ulcerated nipples. Ulcers superficial and readily bleeding. Ulcers may be spreading and deeply penetrating.

Phyt: Nipples sore, sensitive and fissured; intense pain when the child nurses; pain radiated over the whole body.

Puls: Mother weeps every time the child is put to breast; pain extends into chest, neck or down back; shifts from place to place.

Silic: "Nipples ulcerate very easily, are sore and tender; pain in small of back while child nurses."

SORE MOUTH, APTHAE

Apthae mean small whitish ulcers on the surface mucous membrane. Apthae may be on tongue, gums, lips etc.

Therapeutics Leading Indications

Arsen: Livid, bluish. May be white. Gangrenous. Want of appetite and hunger. Burning in mouth.

Borax: Apthae in the mouth inside of cheeks and on tongue, which bleed easily. Great heat and dryness of mouth. Painful red blisters on tongue. Forepart of palate shriveled, paining *esp.* when chewing. Child cries when nursing.

Merc-s: Sore mouth with profuse salivation. Saliva dribbles from mouth of the child. Gums and cheeks ulcerated. Fetid odour from mouth.

Nit-ac: Apthae usually whitish. Blisters and ulcers on tongue. Pricking pain as it from a splinter. Profuse salivation; fetid odour from mouth.

Bapt: Putrid sore mouth. Putrid offensive breath. Gums ulcerated, loose, dark red or purple. Salivation.

Bryon: Tongue, lips, mouth very dry, child refuses to nurse until mouth has been mistuned.

Sulph-ac: Apthae on gums which bleed readily. Apthous mouth of infant or mother; gums may bleed readily. Ulcers spread rapidly in mouth. "Ulceration of mouth, gums, or entire buccal cavity." Profuse salivation.

Ulcer with exceedingly tenacious mucus in mouth: Hydras. Tip of tongue sore: Phyt., Lach. When indicated remedy or remedies fail to cure a case completely: Sulph. Painful excrescences on interior of cheeks: Staph. On inner side of cheeks: Nit-ac., Phyt.

SORE THROAT, PHARINGITIS

Affections of throat attended with pain and inflammation; sometimes with difficulty in swallowing.

Therapeutics Leading Indications

Acon: With characteristic fever of Acon. Burning and picking in throat. Swallowing troublesome.

Apis: Burning, stinging pain when swallowing. Erysipelous louse and oedematous appearance of throat.

Bell: Soft palate highly inflamed and bright red. So may be uvula and tonsils. Inflammation mostly on right side. Deglutition painful or impossible. Swallowing produces spasm of throat.

Hepar: Pricking sensation in throat as from a splinter or fish-bone. Pain relieved by heat. The patient is very sensitive to cold.

Lach: Fauces Purplish, Swollen or ulcerated. Throat feels constricted. Fluid escapes through nose on attempting to swallow. Burning in throat. Swallowing of liquids more painful than solids. All symptoms worse on left side. *Pains worse from drinks. *Worse after sleep.

Merc-s: After Bell. When is cannot effect further improvement. Uvula swollen and elongated. Mouth full of saliva yet throat feels very dry. Constant inclination to swallow. Swallowing of liquids difficult, which are frequently forced back through nose. Tonsils dark red and studded with ulcers.

All-c: Sore throat with coryza which is profuse and acrid, lachrymation being non-excoriating. Cold sensation in throat.

Bryon: Great dryness of throat. Stitching pain when swallowing. Motion increases pain. Constipation.

Bapt: Fauces dark red, studded with dark putrid ulcers which are painful. Odour from mouth very offensive. Solids cause gagging, can swallow only liquids.

Canth: Burning sensation in throat, throat feels 'on fire'. Throat inflamed and covered with plastic lymph.

Dulc: Sore throat caused by cold change of weather.

Lac-c: Throat has glistening red patches of China whiteness; silvery shiny deposits: or glistening red patches. While swallowing pains in throat extend to ears. Sore throat begins and ends with menstruation (Mag-c). Pains first felt on one side then on the other.

Rhus-t: Throat feels stiff after straining. Sensation of dryness in throat. Sticking or stinging pains which are worse on beginning to swallow. Glands under ears much swollen.

Chronic Sore Throat

Alumin: Chronic dryness of throat. Soreness, hoarseness, and great dryness of throat. Thick and sticky mucus may accumulate in throat, expectoration being difficult. Relief from taking anything warm. Clergyman's sore throat.

Arg-n: Of those who use their voices much, as in the case of singers, lecturers, hawkers. High notes cause cough. Chronic hoarseness. Feeling as if something clogged the vocal cords. Sensation of a splinter in throat, felt more on swallowing (Hepar, Nit-ac., Silic.).

Arnic: Great hoarseness and sore throat from excessive use of voice.

Caust: *Soreness and rawness of throat. Hoarseness with rawness. Burning pains in throat with *soreness.

Kali-bi: Chronic congestion of throat. Secretion of stringy mucus from posterior nares. Throat pains more when tongue is put out.

Nat-m: Throat feels very dry, yet the patient constantly hawks up transparent, thin mucus. Sensation of constriction in throat.

Phyt: Pain in eating or drinking things. Dryness in the throat.

SPERMATORRHEA AND POLLUTIONS

Pollution means involuntary discharge of semen with more or less orgasm. It generally occurs at night and very rarely during the day. Nocturnal pollutions generally take place between the years of sixteen and twenty-five, and are not generally harmful when they do not occur more than once a week.

Spermatorrhoea consists of an involuntary discharge of seminal fluid without orgasm, occurring either at stool, on emission of urine, on movements, on the least excitement, after the most trivial erection or even without any cause. Self-abuse frequently results in spermatorrhoea and nocturnal pollutions. Which in their turn bring on impotence.

Therapeutics Leading Indications

Calc-c: Frequent emissions at night which debilitate both mind and body. Weak in legs, weak in ankles, weak in back, weak in heart and weak all over. Decisively weak after a short walk. Palpitation of heart, giddiness, difficult thinking, weakness of memory and confusion of ideas.

China: Frequent nocturnal emission and great weakness caused thereby. Consequence of excessive seminal losses; of self-abuse. Spermattorrhoea. Pale sickly expression; eyes sunken and surrounded by blue and dark margins; perspiration very profuse and very debilitating *esp.*, at night; sweat's easily on least exertion.

Digit: Nocturnal emissions during sleep. Even without dreams, with great weakness, dejection and palpitation after waking up. A useful remedy in spermatorrhoea.

Gels: Involuntary emission of semen. Sexual power exhausted, slightest caress causes a discharge of semen. Genitals cold and relaxed.

Nux-v: Spermatorrhoea caused by masturbation. Pollutions *esp.* towards morning and fatigue on waking. Digestion impaired. Feels un refreshed or worse in every way soon after waking in morning. Flaccidity on penis during coition. Even harmless words offend the patient.

Phos-ac: Bad effects of pre-pubic masturbation. Discharge of prostatic fluid during stool. Frequent and very debilitating pollutions. Several pollutions in one night. Such losses of semen debilitate both mind and body, and the patient is sad, abashed, and despondent of cure, but all the same, there is irresistible desire to masturbate. The patient is greatly distressed by the culpability of the act. Seminal emission when straining at stool. Weak feeling in chest, from talking. Frequent urination.

Sulph: Spermatorrhoea and nocturnal pollutions of morbid nature have often their foundation on sporic constitution and that is way a dose of Sulph. 30 or 200 even. When it is not indicated as it should be, often has the effect of obliterating the tendency to masturbation, and goes a great way towards curing these disorders. Sulph. Itself has frequent nocturnal pollutions; watery semen. Testes and scrotum are relaxed and they hung flabbily down. Penis cold; coition when attempted is practically a failure, semen escaping too soon.

Thuja: A great remedy for nocturnal seminal emissions. Mother tincture of Thuja in five to seven-drop doses, has the reputation of controlling nocturnal seminal emissions, better than any other remedy, seminal emission awake him.

Agnus: Speratorrhoea in old sinners. Penis small, cold and flaccid. Extreme absence of mind. Nocturnal pollutions even after sexual intercourse.

Agnus: Joints easily twisted. Pains as if dislocated in joints. Sprains being the bad results from over lifting. Feet turn under when walking.

Amm-c: Pains, as of dislocation, drawing and tension of joints as from contraction of tendons.

Graph: Easily injured by lifting. Tendency to strain the back. (Stiffness and complete inflexibility of joints, which may be traceable to strains or sprains.)

Mill: Effects of over lifting or overexertion. Bad effects from sprains (and also from a fall from a height).

STAMMERING

To stammer is to "speak (habitually or on occasion from embarrassment etc.) with halting articulation, *esp.* with rapid repetitions of same syllable", while to stutter is to " keep repeating parts, *esp.* Initial consonants, of words in effort to articulate."

Therapeutics Leading Indications

Bell: Heaviness, trembling, and paralytic weakness of tongue, with difficult and stammering speech. Loss of speech.

Bovis: "Stuttering, *esp.* when reading, unable to utter some words."

Bufo: Stuttering and stammering, angry when not understood.

Cann-s: When stammerers at times suffer from embarrassed speech; at one time words are wanting; at another voice fails.

Caust: Stuttering. Embarrassed and very indistinct speech. Distortion of mouth and tongue when speaking. "he often pronounces words wrong and transposes letters and syllables; stuttering in words rich in consonants; lisping, paretic state of tongue and lips." (**Lilienthal**). Stammering from childhood.

Cicu: Speech embarrassed. He is seized with slight jerking of the head backwards while speaking, *esp.* after uttering a few words freely.

Kali-br: Slow and difficult speech after waking. Disturbances of speech originating in brain. Finds it difficult to collect his thought.

Lac-c: When talking is a very difficult job.

Merc-s: Rapid and stammering speech. Dreadful stammering.

Secale: Stammering, indistinct, weak speech, as it tongue were paralyzed; or as if there is some resistance to be overcome.

Spig: "Repeats the first syllable of the first word several times: after that speaks plainly; helminthiasis."

Stram: Stammering, speech being difficult and unintelligible. Exerts himself a long time before he can utter words. Makes a great effort to speak. Distorts the face.

STYE

Small inflammatory tumor near the edge of eyelid.

In the beginning of most of the cases styes disappear promptly under the action of Pulsatilla alone or in alternation with Aconite. Puls, has stye on upper eyelid with itching, burning and swelling of lids. Puls. Is relieved by cold application. Stye with burning relieved by hot fomentation yield to Arse. With Hepar there is inflammation with great sensitiveness to touch and relief from heat: Staph. Has stye which does not suppurate and break, but remains as a hard nodule. Thuja is another remedy for hardened sties and when there are violent burning and stinging in the lids and profuse lachrymator.

Herring says that should indurations remain after the administration of Staph., Calc-c., or Sepia is to be given after a week or two.

Remedies to prevent reappearance of styes are: Graph., Psor., Hepar., Silic., Sepia., Staph., Sulph.

Styes on or affecting

Upper lid: Bell., Merc-s., Staph Sulph., Puls.

Lower lid: Graph., Phos., Puls., Rhus-t.

Inner Canthi: Nat-m.

Towards inner canthi: lach., Lyco., Nat-m, Puls., Silic. Right upper lid; Amm-c.

Corner of eye: Nat-m., Stan., Sulph.

SUNSTROKE

Sudden falling down, as it struck by apoplexy, being affected by heat, for instance, from exposure to sun's rays, in a crowded place, in hot air, and the like. Apply lukewarm water on head, chest, spine and limbs. Very cold water is injurious.

Leading remedies to prevent Sunstroke

For great thirst; flushed face; dry, hot skiing: Acon.

For great thirst with dry lips and tongue and aversion to motion: Bryon.

For giddiness as if intoxicated as if he would fall down, frequent urination, languidness, dimness of vision and trembling: Gels.

For fatigue, dizziness, Dryness of throat, hoarseness, drowsiness and oppression of breathing: Lach.

Those who are easily affected by the ultra-violet rays of the sun which is so very active on high mountains should take a dose of Lach. 200. Such patients easily get long-lasting headache after such an exposure. I say this from my own experience.

Treatment during an attack

Acon: When head has been exposed to direct rays of the sun, *esp*. when asleep, excessive thirst; redness of eyes and face; anxiety, *restlessness, *fear of death.

Arnic: Heat and burning of head with absence of heat from body (which is cool). Suddenness of attack. Involuntary discharge of stool and urine. Blood-shot eyes.

Bell: First stage of sunstroke. Severe throbbing headache worse when stooping.

Camph: * Sudden and complete prostration of vital forces with great coldness of surface. Body bathed in cold sweat, *esp*. head and neck. Cramps in muscles.

Cels: When headache is much pronounced in occiput marked prostration. Confused. Trembling.

Glon: Violent throbbing headache; brain feels as if expanding. Nausea and vomiting of cerebral origin.

Opium: Unconsciousness; *great soper; *stertorous breathing; dark-red bloated face; eyes half-closed; skin covered with hot sweat. Titanic rigidity.

Amly-n: Intense surging of blood to head. Throbbing in head; bursting out feeling in ears. *Deep facial flushing. Longing for fresh air. Tremor of limbs.

Cactus: Violent congestion coming on suddenly. Heat in head; hands and feet cold. Head feels as if it would burst. Prostration.

Therid: Most unbearable headache, nausea and vomiting; worse from least motion of head. Vision may be lost or everything may seem far off; cannot bear least noise.

Treatment of after-effects

Lach: Chronic after-effects. Sun's heat makes him languid, dizzy, faint; it produces headache.

Nat-c: One of the most prominent remedies for chronic after-effects of sunstroke. With the return of hot weather, suffers from headache. Great debility form heat of summer. Inability to think, feels stupefied in the sun.

Nat-m: Hot weather fatigue, makes him languid, dizzy, faint. Anaemic and cachectic persons.

Selen: Hot weather fatigues. Strength and energy are on the increase as the sun sinks down. Strong inclination to sleep from sheer exhaustion caused by heat, yet he is always worse after sleep. Giddiness in sun-light; Agar. Loss of memory; Anac. Well known streets seem strange to the patient: Glon.

SYPHILIS

The first stage comprises chancre (syphilitic sore) on penis and the bubo arising there from. After two or three months (if not properly treated) the specific ulcer as well as the bubo heal or is rather absorbed in the system. Then comes on the secondary stage characterized by symptoms of a constitutional character, such as febrile disturbance, debility, headache, such as febrile disturbance, debility, headache, sore throat, cutaneous eruptions, alopecia, pain in joints and bones. If the disease is not cured or at least checked by appropriate treatment during the first year of its progress, it is apt to manifest itself in its tertiary form, even after so long a period as forty years after the secondary stage is over. The intervening period may be one of perfect health.

The tertiary form is characterized by the formation of tumors called 'gummata', which most frequently make their appearance in the periosteum, testes, liver and brain. So far as homoeopathic treatment of syphilis is concerned, the term 'tertiary' serves no purpose and so far as diagnosis is concerned it creates confusion.

Lastly a few words about the two kinds of syphilis.

Soft chancre	Hard chancre
Profuse discharge of pus is contagious.	Little or no pus is discharged, the discharge being thin and fluidic.
As a rule many ulcers from which may multiply themselves by auto-inoculation.	Generally one ulcer forms, but if a number of ulcers form, such ulcers from the beginning.
Ulcer usually very painful.	Ulcer not painful.
May become phagedenic.	Very rarely becomes phagedenic.
In bubo, generally and inguinal gland is affected. The bubo develops rapidly and is large.	A number of glands in the inguinal region is involved. The glands feel like a row of flattened peas under the skin.
Bubo always suppurates.	Bubo seldom suppurates.
No constitutional symptom follows.	Constitutional symptoms appear.
Leaves no constitutional taint. Consequently progeny does not inherit the disease in any form.	Hereditary but at a late of tertiary stage, as a rule, healthy children are born to syphilitic parents.

Therapeutics Leading Indications

Mer-s: The king of anti-syphilitic remedies. In the beginning: ulcer (chancre with averted red edges) and a *lardaceous or cheesy bottom. Hard chancre with lardaceous base. Superficial ulceration or spreading and deeply penetrating ulcers. Chancres bleed readily;

very painfully; discharge yellowish, fetid. Secondary stage; sore throat; nocturnal bone pains; round, copper-colured and red spots on skin. Fever originating in syphilis. Syphilitic rheumatism. Syphilitic chronic nasal catarrh, acrid, offensive discharge of green mucus; bones of nose swollen and painful.

Merc-bin-iod: Chancre and bubo indolent; bubo discharging for years. Hard chancre. Bubo from hard chancre. Hard, red swelling in front of prepuce and painless and hard chancres in centre. Swelling of glands in different parts of the body; gums swollen, very tender. "It acts well in old cases of syphilis, particularly in persons of lax fiber, scrofulous, and those who have taken much mercury." Syphilitic eruptions.

Merc-proto-iod: Hard chancre: when given without delay may prevent secondary symptoms. Painless chancres with great swelling of inguinal glands, without tendency of suppurate. *N.B.* hard chancres are particularly amenable to this remedy and merc-bin iod.

Merc-cor: Chancres spread with great rapidity. *Chancre with corroding and acrid pus. Excoriation often leads not only to much-spreading ulcers. But eating away of parts and even perforation producing what is called phagedenic ulcer. Burning is often present. Such ulcers ooze corroding and acrid pus. Syphilitic ulcer perforates nasal septum.

Nit-ac: A great remedy in syphilis occupying perhaps the place next to Merc-s. Often called for when Merc-s. Fails. A typical Nit-ac. Ulcer (Chancre) is offensive, irregular in outline, having zigzag edges. Looks like raw flesh at its base, is deeper than Merc-s. Ulcer, which is rather superficial. Spreads more in circumference than in depth. Base looks like raw flesh. Chancre extremely sensitive to touch. Filled with exuberant granulations which readily bleed from slight touch and when dressing it. *Pricking splinter-like pains in chancres. Syphilitic ulcer in mouth. *Esp.* useful after abuse of mercury. Urine very offensive. Laryngitis in old syphilitic subjects. Syphilitic nodes on tibia with nightly pains.

Kali-iod: *Esp.* called for in tertiary syphilis. When gummatous tumors involve the nervous tissues. Also in chancre with hard edges and curdy pus. Deep-eating chancre. Extensive swelling of glands with paraphimosis. Sensitive syphilitic nodes. Severe bone pains, *esp.* at night; tertiary syphilis. Hard nodules on skull with severe pain or headche.

Badi: Very useful in indurate syphilitic buboes, *esp.* when they have been maltreated (carb-an.). Infantile syphilis, whole convolutes of hard glandular swellings, buboes.

Carb-an: Bubo as hard as stone. Neglected syphilitic buboes as hard as stone. Regarding these Farrington says: "Carbo animalis is especially useful when these have been opened too soon, or when there is a gaping wound which has partly healed, leaving the surrounding tissues of an almost stony hardness." Indurations of exiallary gland from syphilis. Coppery red eruptions or blotches *esp.* on face.

Carb-v: Constitutional syphilis. Syphilitic cachexia. Great debility and emaciation. Characteristic dyspeptic symptoms. Great foulness of all secretions Air hunger.

Hepar: *Esp.* useful after abuse of mercury. Ulcers very sensitive to contact; easily bleeding. Suppuration of bubo. Discharge from ulcers smells like old cheese. Sticking or pricking pain in chancre indicated both Hepar and Nit-ac. Both remédies are equally sensitive to touch. (But what is distinctly characteristic of Nit-ac. Is its bleeding.)

Lach: Chancre which was extremely sensitive to slightest touch of say, cloth of bandage while tight bandaging itself elicited no sensitiveness. Such as case cured radically with a single dose of Lach. 200. Lachesis has gangrenous and phagedenic chancre. Ulcer is surrounded by a bluish areola. Caries of tibia, surrounding parts sensitive and livid. Syphilitic aphonic.

Lyco: Indolent chancre. Syphilitic ulcers on legs sluggish and refuse to heal. Copper coloured eruptions on fore head (Carb-an.). Nervous and weakness.

Phyt: In my hands it has acted like magic in syphilitic eczema of face in a number of cases. Syphilitic rheumatism.

TETANUS AND TRISMUS

Tetanus is characterized by spasmodic contraction of voluntary muscles which may be either general or partial and the body is jerked backward and is bent like a bow (opisthotonos), or forwards (emprosthotonos), or may be perfectly rigid (tonic spasm). Opisthotonos is the form that is most frequently met with. At first the nape of the neck becomes stiff and swallowing becomes difficult. Gradually trimus or lockjaw takes place, under which condition the patient is unable to open the mouth fully and swallowing becomes still more difficult.

In some cases the corners of the mouth may be drawn up (risus sardonicus).

Tetanus is caused by a kind of bacillus which gains entrance into the body through any wound or injury, no matter how slight it may be.

Quite a number of cases can be aborted by the timely administration of Aconite and Hypericum.

Therapeutics Leading Indications

Acon: May abort the disease when there is fever, anxiety, rigidity in muscles of jaws of neck, tingling and numbness. In the beginning of traumatic tetanus. Rigidity of muscles of jaws and neck; body bent backwards; distortion of eyes; frequent alternation of redness and paleness of face; tingling, numbness ; fever, anxiety.

Cicu: Lockjaw and tetanic rigidity from injuries inflicted upon head and spinal column. Convulsions with loss of consciousness and frightful distortion of limbs and whole body; opisthotonos; sudden rigidity, then jerks and violent distortions and then utter prostration. Tonic spasms renewed by slightest touch; from opening door or loud talking (Stram.). Great oppression of breathing.

Hydr-ac: Titanic spasms persistent and tonic. Muscles of face, jaws and back are particularly affected. Ricinus sardonicus. Trismus. Breathing is embarrassed; and thrown back. Face flushed, bluish. Blueness and coldness of surface; pulse feeble, imperceptible; foaming at month. Characteristic notes: 1. Sudden attack and rapid establishment of the disorder. 2. Opisthotonos. 3. Bluish hue. 4. Coldness.

Hyper: A valuable remedy in tetanus after traumatic injuries. *Esp*. indicated in punctured wounds with pointed instruments etc., which if treated with Hyper. 30 internally, tetanus or trismus cannot develop. Even when after sometime violent shooting pains running up limbs make their appearance, Lockjaw and tetanus are evidently impending in most cases. At this stage Hyper. Works wonders. Even when stiffness of neck, lockjaw and lastly tetanus are brought about by a lacerated or punctured would, Hyper. Still acts effectively.

Nux-v: Spasm with tetanic rigidity with bending of body backwards at intervals of a few minutes during which muscles are relaxed; full consciousness during spasms. Extreme rigidity of limbs with great hardness of muscles. Spasms renewed by slightest touch.

Agnus: Attacks of tetanic excited mostly by touch, by drinking and by noise. Cheeks and lips blue; breathing labored during spasms, groaning and closing of eyes, lips wide open, drawn up and down exposing teeth; trismus. Also in tetanus characterized by spasmodic twitching or jerking of muscles. Such tetanus may be of traumatic origin or otherwise.

Arnic: Traumatic tetanus; hot head, cold body, internal chilliness with external heat. General prostration of strength.

Bell: Throws body forwards and backwards; bending of body sideways (pleurothotonous), *esp*. to left. Clenched teeth with painful stiffness of muscles of mastication; involuntary discharge of stool and urine.

Cup-m: Jaws closed with loss of consciousness, foam at mouth, redness of eyes; body bent forward; rigidity of whole body. Opisthotonos. Head bent back-wards Urine escapes. Face bluish.

Passiflora incarnate: (Mother tincture or 1X). Useful in tetanus in hot countries.

Stram: Convulsions excited by sight of bright and dazzling objects and touch. Eyes wide open, rolling and squinting. Lockjaw.

Strychnine: Slightest noise or jar excites spasms. Violent electric-like shocks through the limbs followed by opisthotonos; breathing difficult.

TETANUS NEONATORUM

By this is meant tetanus in newborn babies.

Acon: (May be tried at first). As for symptoms, refer to Acon. Elsewhere in this article.

Arnic: When head alone or face alone is hot, while the rest of the body is cool.

Bell: Is often called for, as for symptoms of comes after to the remedy toward the beginning of this stage. A special symptom is: Sudden jerks and shrikes deep.

Camph. Already dealt with. Great coldness on face and head.

Cicu: Symptoms already noted.

Opium: Screams before and during a spasm eyes half open. Rigidity of whole body, the truly turned in the form of an arch.

These are the principal remedies.

TONGUE, DISCOLOURATION OF

The following hints will be of great use in the selection of remedies in various kinds of diseases. Needless to add that a medicine can hardly be selected on the basis of a single tongue indication, but then such an indication helps much in finding out the right remedy in any particular case. But then, certain tongue symptoms are highly characteristic, and the remedy indicated by any one of them is in almost all cases the right remedy, which will be found to be called for by other symptoms of the case as well. How this happens is a mystery of the subtle science of Homoeopathy.

Highly Characteristic Tongue Symptoms

A dry or dark coated tongue *with a red triangular lip: Rhus-t. A white yellowish tongue with *a red streak down the middle: Ver-v.

*Thick, Milky-white coating: Ant-c.

Thick, Yellow coating at the base: Merc-proto-iod.

*Swollen, flabby tongue which takes the imprint of teeth: Merc-s. Red stripe down the centre: Caust, Ver-v.

As if painted white: Arsen.

Deep longitudinal cracks on tongue: Syph.

Fairly Characteristic Ones

A black coating: Arsen., Carb-v., Chin., Merc-s. Ver-a. Bluish tongue: Mur-ac.

Brown: Arsen., Bapt., Hyos., Lach., Phos., Rhus-t., Secale. Green: Nat-s.

Red edges: Arsen.,Mer-s., Sulph.

Lead coloured: Arsen.

Milk-white coating: Glon.

White coating only on one side: Rhus-t.

A white streak on both sides: Caust.

Yellow coating at base: Kali-bi.

TONSILITIS QUINSY

Inflammation of a tonsil of both tonsils and subjacent mucous membrane of the throat.

Therapeutics Leading Indications

Apis: Red and highly inflamed tonsils. Dryness in mouth and throat, without thirst. *Stinging-burning pain when swallowing. Ulcers on tonsils and palate with oedematous appearance around ulcers. Worse from heat and better from cold.

Bar-c: Tonsils tend to suppurate, *esp*. the right. Liability to quinsy after cold. Removes predisposition to quinsy. Pain in throat worse from empty swallowing; pricking sensation when swallowing; swelling of palate; sensation of a plug in throat, worse when swallowing solids. Useful in tonsilitis of infants. *Esp.* adapted to scrofulous, dwarfish children. (*N.B.* if given early before suppuration take place, it will disperse the swelling.) Chronic indurations of tonsils (Lyco.).

Bell: Tonsils swollen, inflamed, of a bright red colour. Worse on right side. Great dryness of fauces and throat, During swallowing, sensation in the throat as if it were too narrow. Ulcers form rapidly on tonsils.

Hepar: When there is a tendency to frequent recurrence of the disease. Chronic tonsillitis accompanied by hardness of hearing. *Sensation as it a fish-bone or a splinter was sticking in throat. Stitching pain in throat extending to ear. Very sensitive to cold air.

Lach: *Esp.* left sided tonsillitis. Throat purplish; inability to swallow; choking when swallowing; or when swallowing, pain extends from the throat right up to the ear. Liquids cause more difficulty in swallowing than solids. Symptoms begin to get worse at 4 p.m. and after sleep.

Merc-s: Tonsils swollen, inflamed and dark blue become ulcerated or studded with ulcers. Swallowing painful. Pain on empty swallowing. Salivation painful sweat without any relief. Quinsy with stinging pain, pus has formed it hastens suppuration.

Silic: Tonsillitis of a severe type. Silic. 12X trit. It said to be almost a specific. Distorts face on each attempt to swallow. Pricking as from pains (stitches) in throat, when swallowing, causing cough. In obstinate cases. When abscesses are forming, yet they do not suppurate *esp.* on left side, or after suppuration, went the suppurating gland I will not heal.

Tuber: Enlarged tonsils. Study the drug under drug Pictures in Silhouette. Many cases of tonsillitis are due to tubercular taint and consequently this remedy is often called for to combat the disease.

Bar-iod: Hypertrophy of tonsils. *Esp.* indicated in chronic enlargement and indurations of tonsils. Swelling of lymphatic glands.

Calc-iod: Chronic tonsillitis. Enlarged tonsils filled with little crypts or pockets.

Kali-m: Acute or chronic tonsillitis when tonsils are covered with whitish coating. Tonsils excessively swollen; stringy tough mucus; swallowing excessively painful, even of water or soft bread; must twist his neck to get it down.

Lyco: Swelling and suppuration of tonsils. Tonsils indurate and studded with many ulcers. Ulceration of tonsils begins on right side. Ulcers in tonsils look like chancre.

TOOTH, DECAYING OF

Therapeutics Leading Indications

Ant-c: Carious teeth with pain at night.

Fluor-ac: Early decay of teeth. Rapid caries of teeth. It favour the expulsion of necroses parts.

Kreos: Teeth decay almost as soon as they appear. Teeth with dark specks thereon begin to decay as soon as they appear. All these decaying conditions of teeth are often associated with spongy, bleeding gums and foul odour from mouth.

Merc-s: Crown of teeth decay, roots remaining intact. Carious. Teeth feel loose, denuded of gums, fall out.

Mezer: Hollow teeth decay very rapidly. Crowns are intact, roots or sides decay (Merc-s. attacks the crown.).

Staph: *Teeth turn black, black streaks run through them and soon crumble. Teeth decay on edges. Blackness, brittleness and caries of teeth. During dentition teeth decay as soon as they are cut. In cases where there is syphilitic and sychotic taint.

Syph: Teeth decay at the edge of gum and break off. Children's teeth are cupped. Teeth have serrated edges. (often a sign of hereditary syphilis).

Thuja: Teeth decay at the roots (sycotic) as soon as they appear, crowns remaining sound. Decay at gums. Crumble and turn yellow.

TOOTHACHE

Toothache may arise from cold, from getting wet, from decayed teeth, from an abscess at the root of a tooth or from some constitutional disorder.

Therapeutics Leading Indications

Acon: The patient is besides himself with pain, or in other words, almost frantic with pain, and Coffee has failed to relieve the pain. Toothache from cold or dry cold winds.

Alumin: As a remedy for toothache, no mention in our therapeutics. Use of Aluminum wares in one of the blunders of modern civilization. Not a few cases of toothache and gum affections can well be traced back to the slow poisoning caused by Aluminum utensils used in cooking food. Alumina in a high potency is supposed to combat the effect there of. Alumina is particularly called of in toothache when excited by chewing and when pain extends to other parts as far as zygomatic bone (bony arch of cheek), and to forehead and temples. Other symptoms: Piercingly painful carious teeth; ulcerated gums; ulcerated roots of teeth; sensation of elongation of teeth; toothache attended with nervous irritation, as after a chill.

Amm-c: Violent toothache as soon as she goes to bed at night. Teeth painful on biting them together.

Ant-c: After extraction of a tooth; it stops bleeding and accelerates healing of gums.

Arsen: Sharp aching pains in teeth and gum, chiefly at night, sometimes extending to cheek, ear, temple. Pains driving to furious despair. Teeth seem loose and elongated when chewing, sensation as if teeth were being pressed into ulcerated spots. (Another gem. Italics mine. Pain relieved by heat of stove, by hot application, or by sitting up in bed.

Bell: Teeth and gums painfully sensitive. Heat and throbbing. Worse from contact of hot food or liquids.

Bryon: Toothache usually of rheumatic origin and frequently occurs in teeth. Affected tooth feels too long and loose, but is not so. Aggravated by taking anything warm in mouth; also by lying on the painless side.

Carb-v: Obstinate looseness of teeth. Toothache provoked by taking anything cold or hot, or salt food. Particularly useful when gums are spongy and bleed.

Cham: *Esp*. in children. But no adult reaps infinity benefit from it is hundreds of cases when: pains drive the patient to despair; the patient moans; there is hot swelling of checks. Pains occur chiefly at night when warm in bed (Phos-ac.); pains extend into ears at their heights; very irritable and whining mood during pain; with salivation (Dulc., Merc-s.); in sound teeth.

China: Toothache relieved by strong pressure, or by pressing teeth together; a slight touch, however, aggravates the pain excessively. Teeth are loose and painful when chewing. Toothache of nursing mothers.

Clem: Toothache relieved by cold water, or drawing in cold air, worse from heat of bed. Worse from smoking tobacco. From crumb of bread. Slight touch exceedingly painful, with an excessive flow of saliva.

Coff: Unbearable pain which drives the patient almost frantic. The patient weeps, trembles, and does not know what to do. *Pain is relieved by holding ice-cold water in mouth. *N.B.* In maddening pains when Coffee fails given Acon. and when Acon. fails try Ver-a., hyos., Sulph.

Dulc: From taking cold in damp or wet weather. Aggravation always from a cold change in weather.

Hepar: Often useful after bell. And Merc-s. When the painful swelling of gums continues, or for a throbbing pain as if blood were entering or forcing into teeth. Swollen inflamed gums, very painful to slight touch.

Hyos: Toothache driving to despair (Caff., Acon., Ver-a., Sulph.). Pains extend to cheeks and along lower jaw, or from cheeks to forehead.

Kreos: It is wrong to eulogize the 3rd and 30th potency as is often done. The 30th and 200th are equally splendid in results, as I have verified times out of number. Often a single dose is required. When teeth are decayed, *esp.* when gums are scorbutic. Teeth decay rapidly. Bad odour from decayed teeth. Gums bluish red, soft, spongy, bleeding; ulcerated. Pains often extend to temples. (Gels., Mag-c.) Malignancy.

Lach: Pains extend from jaw to ear. *Toothache every morning after awaking. Toothache after dinner everyday. Affects the ears. Worse after hot cold drinks; after eating; *after awaking.

Mag-c: Toothache insupportable while at rest, so that the patient is obliged to get up and walk about at night. Pains extend to temples, with swelling of cheek of affected side. Immediate relief from a cold drink. During pregnancy. In sound teeth. Ailments from cutting wisdom teeth.

Merc-s: Toothache in decayed teeth. Pains often extend to ear. Sometimes painful swelling of cheek, salivation, and shivering. Worse at night; worse from warmth of bed. Renewed by fresh air, as well as by eating or drinking anything either hot or cold, particularly by damp air.

Nat-s: Toothache aggravated by warm things, intolerable by contact with hot things, and better by holding cold water in mouth.

Nux-v: Pain from a decayed tooth affecting whole face and even the bones, or extending over the whole side. Pains extend to head, ears, and molar bones; with painful swelling of submaxillary glands. Pains worse in morning. From cold or cold things; relieved by warmth.

Phos-ac: Hollow teethache only when particles of food get into them; pains go away then they have been removed. Teeth become yellow.

Plantago: Toothache with earache; with salivation. Intolerance of warm room. I have not much faith in Plantago mother tincture which is said to relieve toothache, if applied externally; at least I do not venture to extol its efficacy as others have done in matters relating to its application.

Puls: Toothache worse evening and night; in warmth of the bed; from taking anything warm in mouth. Relieved in open air; from drawing cool air in mouth. Worse when sitting, better when walking about: better from pressure. Pains extend to face, ear, head and eye of the side affected.

Spig: Toothache, so that he was unable to sleep at night; it drove him out of bed. No aching during day except just after eating, it at all. But not while eating.

Rhust-t: Caused by a chill. Frequently insufferable, during night, worse in open air and better by external heat. As if teeth were being pressed into their sockets.

Staph: Best indicated when teeth are black, crumbling, carious; *black streaks run through them. Severe gnawing, tearing pains in decayed teeth; sometimes extending to the ear, with throbbing in temple. Worse after eating and chewing; after drinking anything cold, in open air, during night or towards morning. Frequently relieved by hard pressure.

Thuja: Gnawing pain in decayed teeth, greatly aggravated by contact with cold things, or by mastication. *Decay of root of teeth, crown remaining sound.

Arenea diadema: Toothache worse at night on lying down. Painfulness of all teeth as soon as he goes to bed at night. Toothache everyday at the same hour.

Ignat: "Soreness and tenderness in teeth, felt more in the intervals between than when eating."

TUMOURS

Therapeutics Leading Indications

Tumours containing morbid matter: Apis, Arsen., Bar-c., Brom., Calc-c., Graph., Heper., Silic.

Such tumour on skull: bar-c.

Intolerable pain in tumour; Stram.

Pricking in tumour: Hepar.

Lancinating pain; Coni.

Wens (more or less permanent tumour benign character on scalp or other parts of body): Bar-c., Bell., Coni., Graph., Kali-c., Nit-ac., Phyt., Silic., and Thuja.

Burning: Bar-c.

Malignant: Crotal.

On knees: Ant-c., Calc-f.

Fibroid tumour of ulcerus; Tereb., Thuj.

Fibroid on os; Ustil.

Malignant tumour of uterus with tendency to hamemorrhage, system being in a degraded state: Crotal.

In vagina Lyco., Puls., silic.

Glandular tumour where no glands are usually found: Lapis albus.

Blusih nodes (hard tumour) on skin: magnum aceticum. Nodes on forehead, tibia and other places; syphilitic taint: Still. Fibroid (of Fibrous structure) tumours of breast: Thyroidinum, Teuc.

Brawny (strong muscular or fibrous swelling 'anywhere: Thyoidimum.

Uterine fibroids: Thyroidinum, Teue.

Lumps (indurated) form on the skin: Sepia.

Fibrous tumours of eyelids, *esp*. inside lower lid; Teue.

Sansitive syphilitic nodes; Kali-i.

Abdominal tumour: Kali-i. (ex).

Womb packed with fibroids: Kali-i.

Lumps and nodules, indurate, under the skin all over body (these may be painful or painless): Bar-c.

Indurations of cartilages about joints: Aur-met.

TYPHOID FEVER

Generally runs a course of three to five weeks, mortality being maximum during the third week. The early symptom of the disease which manifest themselves a few days before an attack are debility, headache, indisposition and sometimes nosebleed. The attack is ushered in by violent chill or slight feverishness followed by high fever. Tenderness or pain on firm pressure in the right side of the bowels (right iliac fassa, near the termination of the small intestine), Gurgling in this region on pressure, a few red spots appearing usually upon the abdomen and chest are a few peculiar symptoms of the disease.

Therapeutics Leading Indications

Arnic: Indifference to everything, wants to be let alone, does not want to be talked to, says there is nothing the matter with him. Disinclined to answer questions. While answering falls into a deep stupor before finishing. Comatose drowsiness with delirium. The whole body feels sore and bruised. Bed feels too hard; tosses about to find a soft place. *Stupor with involuntary discharge of stool and urine. Heat of upper part of body; coldness of lower. Tongue dry with a brown streak down the middle. Horribly offensive stool. Fetid breath. Tympannic distension of abdomen.

Arsen: Indicated late in the disease. *Great restlessness and anxiety with fear of death; *extreme prostration; drinks little but often. Lips, gums and teeth covered with black sores. Burning in stomach and bowels, which are sensitive to pressure. All symptoms worse about midnight.

Bapt: In the beginning when there is *bruised, sore feeling all over body. It is also useful in the late stage, when the patient is dull and confused. Heavy sleep, can scarcely be aroused long enough to answer a question.

Bryon: Desire to lie down and remain quiet. *Aversion to least motion. Constant inclination to yawn. This something like that of Gels. Drowsiness with half-close eyes. Light and noises unbearable. Dry lips and mouth with a strong desire for cold drinks. Hasty drinking of cold water. Also hasty speech. *Dizziness of fainting on sitting up.

Carb-v: Mostly in the last stage. Face pale, sunken, Hippocratic; cyanotic blueness of face, lips and tongue. Cold surface, *esp.* below knees to feet; cold knees even when they are covered with bed clothes. Cold sweat on limbs. Voice hoarse or lost. Great foulness of all secretions. Vital forces nearly exhausted.

Gels: In early stages. Extreme prostration in the initial stage; feels sore and bruised all over body; dreads movement on account of weakness. Dull and drowsy. *Eyelids feel heavy, can hardly keep them open. Full dusky-red face. Constant yawning. Little or no thirst. Trembling from weakness. Tongue trembles on attempting to protrude it.

Hyos: In advanced stages. In the early stage, answers question correctly, but stupor and delirium return immediately. This delirium grows more and more profound, until there sets in profound stupor from which the patient cannot be roused. Grasps at flocks (Bell., Bryon., Phos-ac.). Picks at bed clothes (Bell., Stram.). Raises head from pillow and gazes about. Twitching and jerking of limbs.

Lach: Rapid onset, intensity and rapid failure of strength. Face purple, mottled tremor of the tongue, which catches on the teeth when protruded. Fetid breath; fetid excretions. Stupor or muttering delirium; falling of lower jaw.

Mur-ac: Advanced cases. So prostrated that he slides down towards the foot of the bed. The lower jaw hangs down. Sores on teeth. Putrid stool, offensive breath and offensive body smell. Involuntary putrid stool while urinating. Involuntary stool and urine. Bed sores. Nosebleed. Bleeding from the anus. Pulse is intermittent every third beat.

Nit-ac: In advanced stages. *Hemorrhage from bowels; great sensitiveness of abdomen. Extremely offensive urine. Anxiety about recovery, with fear of death. *Esp.* indicated in patient with tubercular history. (Author).

Pyro: When fever commences with pain in limbs, you may at once give this remedy, unless any other remedy is sharply indicated. There is aching all over body feels hard. The patient cannot lie more than a few minutes in one position, feels better by changing position (This state of affairs being due to pain). All secretions and excretions putrid, foul-smelling. Taste sweetish; horribly putrid. Tongue clean, smooth, fiery red as if varnished. Pulse abnormally rapid, being out of all proportion to temperature. Forehead bathed in cold sweat. Cold sweat over whole body.

Apis: Skin is burning hot in some places, while unnaturally cold in others. Skin alternately dry and perspiring. Great drowsiness. Great prostration, the patient slides down in bed. Thirstlessness.

Great bruised soreness and bloodedness of abdomen. Tongue trembles and catches on the teeth while protruding it (Lach.).

Bell: In early stages with symptoms as given under Simple Fever. Also indicated in violent delirium with disposition to bite, tear things etc.

Hamam: Hemorrhage from the bowels of venous blood which is fluid, dark and fetid, without anxiety. Exhaustion out of all proportion to blood lost, yet the patient exhibits no anxiety. Great soreness of abdomen.

Lyco: Stupid with dropped jaw; half-open eyes; one foot (right) hot, the other cold. At the end of the second week when rash fails to appear and the patient becomes unconscious with muttering delirium, picks bed clothes, abdomen becomes distended with gas, flatus rumbles and crooks in the abdomen, in the chest is heard rattling.

Opium: When indicated remedies fail to act. Opium may be given in order to arouse the reactive energies of the system. It is indicated by unconsciousness with half-closed glassy eyes, snoring respiration, body bathed in cold sweat.

Large quantities of coagulated blood passes from anus with extreme weakness: Alumen. Before an attack if there be fear of being crazy or that he will lose his senses: Chlorine. (A few drops of chlorine water may be given as a dose.). Fear of death: Arsen., Bapt, also Bryon., Rhus-t. Dropping of lower jaw; Arsen. Bapt., Carb-v., Lach., Lyco., Restless wants to go from one bed to another: Arsen., also Calc-c., Cina, Cham. Rhus-t.

ULCERS

Therapeutics Leading Indications

Arsen: Ulcer indolent; rather superficial; fetid smell, putridity; burning; apt to bleed easily; better from heat.

Asaf: Ulcers are intolerably sensitive to touch around edges; easy bleeding; pus thin, ichorous and putrid.

Carb-an: Ulcers are indurate. Ulceration of surface or of internal parts; with putrid discharges. Cancerous ulcers. Malignant ulcers with burning pain (Arsen.); readily bleeding.

Hepar: Ulcers of a very low type, flat, rather superficial; very sensitive to touch; readily bleeding; discharge of pus and blood; discharge smelling like old cheese; edges very sensitive; *little pimples surround the principal ulceration.

Kali-bi: It ulcerates, particularly, the mucous membrane. Painful ulcer on tongue. Ulceration of uvula and tonsils. Septum ulcerates. Ulcer of roof of mouth with sloughing (in syphilis). Chronic intestinal ulceration (Merc-s.). Ulcers on previously inflamed feet. Ulceration with thick crust as on glans penis, nasal septum (these being ulcers hidden under scabs). Note that these show no tendency to heal. Ulcers corrode and become deeper and deeper. Deep-eating ulcers. Perforation of septum. Lastly: *punched out (as if cut with a punch) perforating ulcers. Kali-bi. Ulcers are indolent.

Lach: Ulcers: greatly sensitive to touch (but not to pressure); gangrenous; of bluish appearance all round them; of offensive smell. Ulcers with blue surrounding; with many pimples around. Ulcers (on a purple skin) surrounded by pimples, vesicles and other small ulcers.

Merc-s: Superficial, flat; readily bleeding; readily spreading; lardaceous base; margins averted like raw meat. Worse from heat of head and hot and cold applications.

Mezer: Large ulcers surrounded by pustules. Ulcers with thick, yellowish white scab, under which thick pus collects. Easily bleeding, sensitive, painful at night. A honey-like scab around mouth.

Nit-ac: Ulcers and cracks are in particular found around mucous outlets of the body where skin and mucous membrane join. Ulcers bleed easily; offensive; irregular (zigzag) in outline; *pricing pains as of splinters, *esp.* on contact, Nit-ac. Ulcers are often filled with exuberant granulations with readily bleed from slight touch.

Puls: Inflamed on putrid ulcers.

URINARY AILMENT

Therapeutics Leading Indications

Acon: Urination painful, difficult, drop by drop; urine scanty, scalding hot, red or dark-coloured. Retention from cold, *esp*. in children.

Apis: Urine scanty or suppressed; burning, stinging, and soreness when urinating.

Berb: Sensation of pressure on making water. Burning pains in urethra when making water, and afterwards, but *esp*. at other times. Urination accompanied by pains in thigh and loins.

Canth: Retention and suppression of urine. Constant, intolerable urging to urinate. Urine scalds him; passed drop by drop (Acon., Bell.). Discharge of urine is at times attended by so great burning that it could not be worse if the urine were molten lead.

Caust: Paralysis of bladder from long retention of urine. Involuntary urination when coughing, blowing nose or sneezing.

Gels: Incontinence of urine from paralysis of sphinter (Caust.). Tenesmus of bladder.

Lyco: Children often cry out before urinating.

Pareira: Violent pain in glans penis when straining to urinate. Pains down thigh and even to feet when passing water.

Sars: Great pain is experienced near neck of bladder *soon after an emission of urine (that is, just at the end of urination). Can pass urine only when standing; when one sits it dribble. Child screams before and while passing urine.

Retention of urine with full bladder; strangury with tenesmus of the neck of bladder: Camph. Complete retention of urine; urging and straining, but cannot pass a drop: Cann-i. When urinating urethra feels drawn up into knots: Cann-s. Burning when urinating, but *esp*. just after: Cann-s. Inability of pass urine without standing with feet wide apart: Chimaphila. Urine stops suddenly, and does not begin to flow for some moment; Coni. Difficult urination; urine at first flows in full stream then stops, flows again and so on; Coni pressure on bladder if it is too full, not relieved by frequent urination: Digit. Paralysis of bladder with involuntary discharge of urine: Digit. Paralysis of bladder with involuntary discharge of urine: Dulc. Constant desire to urinate, felt deep in abdomen; Dulc. Has to wait awhile before urine passes; flow intermittent; Dulc. Urine passes slowly without force, dropping vertically from urethra without force: Hepar. Retention of urine with pressure in bladder; *esp*. in retention of urine after labour are in lying in women: Hyos. Fetid urine having intolerably offensive strong smell, or smells like horse's urine: Nit-ac. Retention of urine after delivery; retention of urine from fright; Opium. Sudden irresistible urging to urinate with or without Gonorrhoea Petros. Involuntary urination when coughing or walking: Puls. Frequent urging to urinate with profuse emission: Thuja. Flow of urine stops several times before bladder is empty: Coni., Thuja. Dribbling after urination: Thuja. Urging to urinate frequent and hasty: Thuja. Hasten to urinate, must or urine is discharge: Arnic., Canth., Clem., Kroes., Nux-v. Petrasel, Puls., Sepia. Lenconcebus passing of urine: Arg-n., Caust. Wait awhile must, before urine passes: Arnic., Caust., Heper, Lyco., Rhus-t., Sepia.

UTERUS, PROLAPSUS DISPLACEMENT OF

Therapeutics Leading Indications

Agar: Prolapsces after menopause; awfully bearing down pains; almost intolerable.

Aur-met: Uterus enlarged and prolapsed. Weight of organ causing prolapsed, (the ailment is due to chronic congestion of uterus and not due to relaxation of the ligaments). Prolapsus and indurations of uterus.

Bell: In recent cases of prolapsus. Bearing down pains as if everything would protrude through vulva; heat and dryness in vagina; backache with feeling as if back would break.

Calc-c: Prolepsus with sensation of pressure on uterus; bearing down pains worse on standing. General symptoms of the remedy.

Lil-t: *Bearing down sensation, in abdomen and pelvis, as though all organs would escape. Must cross legs to relieve the sensation of bearing down; must place hands to vulva to prevent contents finding its way out of vagina. On rising to walk, uterus falls by its own weight. Prolapsus due to laxity of ligaments.

Murex: Prolapsus of uterus; bearing down sensation, as if the internal organs would be pressed out; must keep legs tightly crossed, to relieve the pressure. *Sore pain in uterus.

Podo: Prolapsus after over lifting of straining, or after delivery; bearing down with sensation as if genitals would come out during stool.

Nux-v: Prolapsus from straining or lifting; pressure towards genitals, *esp.* in morning; frequent ineffectual urging to stool.

Rhus-t: Prolapsus from overexertion of straining; pain in small of back relieved by lying on something hard.

Sepia: Prolapsus of uterus and vagina; feeling of weight, heaviness, with dragging down; as if everything would protrude from pelvis; must cross limbs to prevent protrusion of parts, with oppression of breathing.

Prolapsus: During menopause, with flushes of heat, and heat on top of head: Lach. Caused by concussion. Cannot walk erect: Arnic. With tendency to miscarry: Helon./Worse during stool: Stan.

VARICOSE VEINS

Affected parts bluish, soreness, stinging: Puls.

Veins highly inflamed; swollen: Puls.

Painful: Brom., Caust., Puls. (Worse towards evening).

Stinging pains: Apis.

On legs; Fluor-ac., Hamam., Puls., Lyco.

On legs, Great pain, can scarcely move about: Hamam.

On legs, tending to ulceration: Fluor-ac.

On legs, during pregnancy; with cramping pains at night, preventing sleep: Hamam.

On legs during pregnancy: Arnic., Carb-v., Caust., Fluor-ac., Graph., Hamam., Lyco., Nux-v., Puls.

Swelling of veins to ankles during pregnancy: Lyco.

VERTIGO GIDDINESS

Therapeutics Leading Indications

Acon: Giddiness on rising from a recumbent position may be with vanishing of sight.

Ambr: Vertigo when moving about. *Esp*. in open air, legs unsteady.

Arg-n: With general debility and trembling from nervous weakness.

Bell: On stooping or when rising after stooping. As in objects turned in a circle.

Brom: Excited by seeing running, water, or anything moving rapidly. Relieved by nosebleed.

Bryon: With sensation of looseness in brain when stopping, and when raising up the head. Tendency to reel backward.

Caust: In the incipiency of paralysis. Anxiety, weakness of head, redness of face.

China: From debility from loss of vital fluids.

Coccul: From motion of carriage (Bryon.).

Ferr-m: Excited when rising suddenly from a lying to a sitting posture. When descending a height. Walking over a bridge or by some flowing water causes vertigo.

Graph: After a good sleep, *esp*. on looking upward.

Kali-c: Adapted particularly to the anaenic. On turning head rapidly or from riding in a carriage.

Lach: On closing eyes; with staggering to left side. Early in morning on waking. Frequent momentary vertigo, *esp*. on closing eyes.

Lyco: In morning and after rising. Reels back and forth.

Nat-c: When working in the sun.

Ipec: Intense nausea. Nausea is more characteristic than vomiting. Nausea with profuse salvation. Vomiting without relief. Vomiting of large quantity of flairy mucus. Tongue clean or slightly coated.

Nux-v: Feels very sick at stomach. Nausea, feeling as of vomiting would bring great relief. Nausea in morning.

Puls: Nausea and vomiting with bad taste in mouth. Vomiting of food eaten long ago. Nausea and vomiting *esp.* in evening, or after eating or drinking.

Rhus-t: Vomiting of cerebral origin. Giddiness. Sang: Nausea not relieved by vomiting. Vomiting with craving to eat in order to quiet the nausea. Nausea with headache.

Ver-a: Violent vomiting with excessive nausea, and great prostration, worse from drinking or by least motion. Profuse salivation and violent thirst. *Cold sweat on forehead.

WARTS

Small hard excrescences on the skin. If warts are numerous, they generally heal very rapidly, whereas the isolated ones have at times the tendency to bid defiance to all treatment.

Therapeutics Leading Indications

Caust: Warts large, jagged and bleed easily. Hard, dry, horny warts. Seedy warts. Fleshy warts growing near nails are always cured with Caust. Old warts on nose.

Nit-ac. Warts may itch and prick. Jagged. Syphilitic, elevated, exuberant and cauliflower-like. Also, horny, large, old, pedunculated; soft with thin epidermis and moist. Pricking pain.

Thuja: Wart-like excrescences here and there, *esp.* on hands and genitals. Warts on any part of body with little necks. Warts hard, cleft and seedy. Fan-shaped on genitals. Smelling like old cheese (Hepar). Sycotic moist excrescences on glands, prepuce and arms. Sycotic excrescences on neck of uterus. Warts split easily. May bleed and itch. "Warts and new growths of many kinds." (J.H. Clarke).

Horny warts: Ant-c., Calc-c., Sepia and Thuja. Horny warts on hands: Ant-c. Pedunculated warts: Caust., Dule., Thuja., Also Rhus-t., Lyco. Fleshy Warts: Caust., Dulc., also Rhus-t. Isolated warts: Caust., Caust., Calc-c., Nat-C. Bleeding: Caust., Nit-ac., Thuja., also Cinnam., Rhus-t.

On face: Caust., Dulc., also Nit-ac., Sepia. On neck: Nit-ac. On palms of hand: Anac., Nat-m. On eyelids: Caust. On glans: Nit-ac., Phos-ac., Thuj. Gonorrhoal; Thuja. Smooth, soft; Ant-c. Suppurating: Calc.c.

WHITLOW, FELONS

Inflammation of one of the fingers terminating in suppuration is called panaritium. Whitlow or run-around is a superficial form of this disorder, while a deep-seated variety is known as felon.

Therapeutics Leading Indications

Amm-c: Panaritium; deep-seated periosteal pain (Dios., Silic.). Affects right side most. "I have seen the nightly pain which had deprived the patient of sleep, for several nights, relieved in a few hours, and the morbid. Process stayed at the same time by one or two doses of Ammon. Carb. 500." (Raue).

Anth: Whitlow when sloughing takes place. (When there is terrible burning pain, not relieved by Apis. or Arsen., try Anth.

Apis: Burning, *stinging pain. Pain better from cold application.

Arsen: Panaritium with gangrene; burning like fire; worse ofter midnight.

Dios: Whitlow in early stages: pricking, sharp agonizing pain. Simply apply to the part a piece of linen soaked with a very dilute solution of Dios. 30 and the pain will wear off as if by the touch of a magic wand. This is from my own experience. You may or may not also give a dose or two of the remedy internally. Its action seems to me like that of a specific. Disposition of felons is in itself an indication of the drug.

the first; it would not only prevent the good effect of the former but it would be injurious."

Dulcamara: After repercussion of eruptions or when excited by cold, damp exposure.

Ipecac: Child becomes stiff and purple or blue in face: cough causes gagging and vomiting of phlegm. Wheezing in chest (but this symptom I have never met with in any whooping cough case). Kent says that with Ipecac. There are red face, thirstlessness, violent whooping, with convulsions, with gogging and vomiting of all that the child eats. It is not understood where from Kent got "red face." Every fresh attack sets in with a long-drawn, difficult, howling, sighing inspiration. There may be bleeding from nose.

Kali-bichro: Vomiting of viscid or sticky mucus which can be drawn out in long strings. Expectoration is yellowish and not clear like Coccus cacti, says Farrington.

Paroxysms: Long-lasting—Cup-met., Lobi. Every fifteen or twenty minutes, with occasional intervals, lasting an hour—Coral. Short—Bell. Two in quick sulccession—Merc-sol., Sulph. Two in rapid succession at night, followed by long intervals of rest—Merc-sol. Vioent—Coral. Cupr-m., Dros. Drinking aggravates—Cina. Better by swallowing cold water—Cup-m. Brought on by drinking cold water—Ver-a. Associated with wheezing—Ipec., Dros. Associated with whistling—Cup.m.

WORM, AFFECTIONS OF

These are all based upon or rather engrafted on psoric diathesis and consequently the expelling of worms by some specific drug does not mean a cure. Serious troubles may ensue, sometimes several years after the worms will have been expelled by crude drugs, though the form of the disease that would then manifest itself will vary. 'Kill' psora, if you want to 'kill' worms 'radically', or these parasitic vermin's will find the 'rotten' intestine a 'hot bed' for their continual growth and well-being.

What is required is a prolonged course of anti-psoric treatment so as to remove the taint of psora, and the worms will find their habitation not favourable for their nourishment and, eventually they will of their own accord dislodge themselves. Treat psora and not worms, if you intend to exterminate the latter.

Therapeutics Leading Indications

Acon: Febrile disturbance due to worms. Frequent ineffectual urging to stool, or nothing but stool is passed. Itching at anus with restlessness, worse at night.

Cina: Itching of nose; child rubs or picks nose constantly; bores with fingers into nose. Baby rubs nose on pillow or on shoulder of nurse or mother. Itching of anus; discharge of round or thread worms through anus. Grinding of teeth or chewing motion before the child has teeth, during sleep. Gagging cough in morning on rising. Hungry soon after a meal. Refuses mother's milk. Abdomen hard and distended. Colic around navel. One cheek red, the other pale. Face pale, sickly, with dark rings around eyes. Urine turbid white; milky or semi-solid after standing. Particularly useful in long round worms. Also pin worms with itching of anus.

Spig: Itching and sensation of creeping, tackling in rectum and anus. Sensation as of worm rising in throat; better after eating. Nausea every morning before breakfast, better after eating. Blue rings around eyes. Offensive breath. Colic about navel. Dry hard cough at night. Violent palpitation of heart.

Stan: It stupefies the worms and subsequently any purgative would expel the same. Pain in abdomen or colic in children, better from hard pressure, as when the child is taken on the shoulder when its abdomen gets pressed. Such pain is often due to worms in children. Round worms and even tapewarms are passed by Stan. Nausea after eating; hungry but cannot eat enough, except in evening; stomach feels empty even after eating; hungry but cannot eat enough, except in evening; stomach feels empty even after eating; a pale and sunken countenance, with dark rings around eyes, discharge of mucus from bowels with round worms.

Sulph: Particularly useful after Acon., and Merc-s. Creeping in nose. Creeping and biting in rectum. Frequent passage of round worms or thread worms. Sulph. Is frequently required to complete a cure after other remedy or remedies have played their part. Verminous diathesis (Calc-c., Silic.).

Santonine: (1X trit.) Very useful in expelling round worms. Three doses of the same per day for two or three days may be given.

Calc-c: Is one of the medicines often required after treatment with other indicated remedies, in order to eradicate worm diathesis or hereditary predisposition to worms. Worm troubles with constipation.

Silic: Worm diathesis. See general symptoms elsewhere. Stool of the consistence of pap or like pus; with maw-worms; with tapeworms. Children are sickly, wanting in vital heat and they perspire all over head and have worms. Such children may *cry when kindly spoken to.

MARASMUS

Gradual wasting of the tissues of the body from poor absorption of food. This condition is especially observed in Children.

Therapeutics Leading Indications

Abort: Marasmus of children with marked emaciation, sometimes only lower extremities, or emaciation may first be noticed in legs. *Emaciation begins in lower limbs and gradually spreads upwards (opposite of Lyco., Nat-m., Psor.). Skin flabby, hangs loose. Face wrinkled as if old. (*N.B.* My advice is to administer a single dose of the 200th potency and wait for the result for a month or two. Immature repetition may spoil the broth.)

Acet-a: Wasting and debility. Face pale, waxen, emaciated. *Slow fever, with drenching night sweats.

Argent-n: withered, dried up, old-looking person. A child looks like a withered old man. Progressive emaciation. Scrawny, feeble, dried-up-looking woman (Sec.). Cachetic state.

Arsen: Face is pale, care-worn, wrinkled. Prematurely old, and wrinkled skin. Lips and mouth shrivel and become wrinkled. Cold, clammy perspiration.

Bar-c: Abdomen bloated, while the rest of the body emaciated. Child does not want to play; prefers to sit idly in a corner; *slow inept, backward; stupid, silly look. Withered face.

Calc-c: Greatly enlarged abdomen, too large head, while the limbs and neck are emaciated. Emaciation (with swollen abdomen) without failure of appetite. Weakness in legs, in neck, in back, in lungs, in heart, and all over. Averse to exercise, wrinkled face, hair dry.

Calc-p: Children emaciated with sunken, flabby abdomen. Great emaciation, child looking old and wrinkled. Skin dry and cold. Neck too slender, does not support head. Child cannot hold head up, and nurse is obliged to support it.

Hydras: Cachectic or malignant dyserasia with defective assimilation and marked derangement of liver function. Emaciation as well as prostration. Obstinate constipation. No desire for stool for days. Backache.

Iod: Eats ravenously, yet emaciates. Emaciation of single parts. Emaciation progresses to such an extent that the patient is in the long run reduced to the state of a skeleton, although appetite is found good all the time. Enlargement of all glands. Iod. Has also curvature and distortion of bones. Sweats easily and easily becomes exhausted. Always feels to hot.

Nat-m: Emaciated. Dropsical. Malarial cases sea. Losing flesh while living well. Face pale, Shining but not good looking, upper lip swollen. *General emaciation, muscles marked about the neck, which is very thin and shrunken. "The coldness become prominent, and the neck looks scrawny and the hip and lower limbs remain plump and round." (Aryent.) From worms: Cina. In cholera infantum: Arsenic dentition: Ars. In children who are bottle fed: Nat. Mature senility: Con. Incipient: Cham.

RICKETS, RACHITIS

It is a constitutional disease in childhood, characterized by disordered ossification (formation of bone). What are generally noticed are softness and curvature of bones. Largeness of head, enlargement of the joint-ends, *esp.* of the wrists and ankles, voracious appetite, profuse perspiration about head, diarrhoea etc. Mental faculties are amazingly precocious.

Therapeutics Leading Indications

Calc-c: Curvature *esp.* of spine and long bones; extremities deformed and crooked. Swelling and softening of bones. One bone is deplorably deficient in calcium while another manifest abnormal accumulation and develops bony growths. Difficulty in walking and standing and not exactly "difficulty in learning to walk or stand" as H.C. Allen has given in his Keynotes. Out of breathe from slight exertion. Milk disagrees; sour vomiting of large curds.

Calc-p: Tendency of bones to bend and curve. Curvature of spine, with tendency to bend to the left. Bones soft and thin. *Cranial bones (*esp.* occipital) very soft and thin, crackling like paper upon pressure. *Fontanel's remain open too long; may close and reopen. Posterior fontanels very large (Calc-c.) has anterior fontanelle open). See also Marasmus. Slow to comprehend.

Silic: Limbs are shrunken, eyes sunken, face pinched and old-looking; rachitic; emaciated; or stunted growth; body emaciated, while the abdomen is distended, which is hard and may be hot; large-headed with open fontanel's; whole body is wasted, while the head is exceedingly large; *profuse sour-smelling head-sweat,' while the body is dry; spine week; ankles week.

Bar-c: Scrofulous, dwarfish children; imperfect development; cowardly, bashful, timid; afraid of an aversion, to strangers.

Sulph: Distortion (curvature of spine). Vertebrae softened. Cracking of vertebrae on bending head backward. Standing is the most disagreeable position. See Sulphur in drug-pictures.

Name of Medicines

1. Abies Canadensis
2. Abies Nigra
3. Abrotanum
4. Absinthium
5. Acetic Acid
6. Aconitum Napellus
7. Adrenalin
8. Aesculus Hippocastainum
9. Aethusa Cynapium
10. Agaricus Muscarius
11. Agnus Castus
12. Alfalfa
13. Allium Sativum
14. Allium Sepa
15. Aloe
16. Alumina
17. Ambra Grisea
18. Amly Nitrosum
19. Ammonium Bromatum
20. Ammonium Carb
21. Ammonium Muriaticum
22. Ammonium Phosphoricum
23. Anacardium Angelica
24. Anthracinum
25. Antimonium Crudum
26. Antimonium Tartaricum
27. Apis Mellifica
28. Aralia Racemosa
29. Aranea Diadema
30. Argentum Nitricum
31. Arnica
32. Arsenicum Album
33. Arsenicum Iodatum
34. Arsenicum Sulfuratum
35. ASF
36. Asparagus Officinalis
37. Aurum Metallicum
38. Aurum Muriaticum
39. Bacillnum
40. Badiaga
41. Baptisia
42. Baryta Carb
43. Belladonna
44. Benzoic Acid
45. Berberis Vulgaris
46. Bismuthum

47. Borax
48. Bromum
49. Bryonia
50. Bufo
51. Cactus
52. Calcarea Arsenica
53. Calcarea Carbonica
54. Calcarea Fluorica
55. Calcarea Iodata
56. Calcarea Sulphurica
57. Cannabis Sativa
58. Cantharis
59. Capsicum
60. Carbo Vegetabilis
61. Cardus
62. Caulophyllum
63. Causticum
64. Chamomilla
65. Chelidonium Majus
66. Cholesterinum
67. Cicuta Virosa
68. Cina
69. Cinchona Officinalis or China
70. Cinnamonum
71. Cistus
72. Clematis
73. Cobalt
74. Cocculus
75. Colchicum
76. Colocynthis
77. Condurango
78. Conium
79. Cuprum Metallicum
80. Digitalis
81. Dioscorea Villosa
82. Drosera
83. Dulcamara
84. Echinacea Rudbeckia
85. Eupatorium Perfoliatum
86. Eupatorium Purpureum
87. Euphorbium
88. Euphrasia
89. Fel Tauri
90. Ferrum Iodatum
91. Ferrum Metallicum
92. Ferrum Phosphoricum
93. Fluoricum Acidum
94. Fraxinus Americana
95. Gelsemium
96. Ginseng
97. Glonoine
98. Gnaphlium
99. Gossypium
100. Graphites
101. Guaicum
102. Hamamelis Virginica
103. Hekla Lava
104. Helianthus
105. Hepar Sulphonicum (Hippoz)
106. Hydrastis
107. Hydrocyanic Acid
108. Hyoseyamus
109. Hypericum
110. Ignatia
111. Iodum
112. Ipecacuanha
113. Iris Versicolor
114. Jaborande

115. Jonosia Asoca
116. Kali Arsenicum
117. Kali Bichromicum
118. Kali Bromaytum
119. Kali Carbonicum
120. Kali Muriaticum
121. Kali Nitricum
122. Kali Phosphoricum
123. Kali Sulphuricum
124. Kreosotum
125. Lachesis
126. Lachnantes
127. Lapis Albus
128. Ledum
129. Lobelia Inflata
130. Lycopodium
131. Magnesia Carbonica
132. Magnesia Muriatica
133. Magnesia Phosphorica
134. Magnesia Sulphurica
135. Malandrinum
136. Medorrhinum
137. Mercurius Hydrargyrum
138. Mercurius Sulphuricus
139. Mezereum
140. Millefolium
141. Murex
142. Muriaticum Acidum
143. Natrum Carbonicum
144. Natrum Muriaticum
145. Natrum Phosphoricum
146. Natrum Sulphuricum
147. Nitricum Acidum
148. Nux Vomica
149. Opium-Papaver Somniferum
150. Oxalicum Acidium
151. Pareira Brava
152. Passiflora Incarnata
153. Phosphoricum Acidum
154. Phosphorus
155. Physostigma
156. Phytolacca
157. Pilocarpus Microphyllus
158. Plantago
159. Plumbum Metallicum
160. Podophyllum
161. Pothos Foetudus
162. Prunus Spinosa
163. Psorinum
164. Pulsatilla
165. Pyrogenium
166. Ranunculus Bulbosus
167. Ratanhia
168. Rhododendron
169. Rhus Toxicodendron
170. Robinia
171. Rumex
172. Ruta Graveolens
173. Sabadilla
174. Sabina
175. Sambucus Nigra
176. Sanguinarina Nitrica
177. Sarsaparilla
178. Secale Cornutum
179. Selenium
180. Senega
181. Sepia
182. Silicea

183. Silicon
184. Solidago Virga
185. Spigelia
186. Spongia Tosta
187. Stannum
188. Staphysagria
189. Sticta
190. Stramonium
191. Sulphur
192. Sulphur Iodatum
193. Symphytum
194. Tellurium
195. Thlaspi Bursa
196. Thuja Occidentalis
197. Thyrodinum
198. Titanium
199. Trombidium
200. Tuberculinum
201. Urtica Urens
202. Uva-Ursi
203. Variolinum
204. Veratrum Album
205. Verbascum
206. Wyethia
207. Zincum Metallicum
208. Zingiber